Free From Fear

Living Well After Cancer

If you've had cancer, you're probably familiar with the slow, creeping fear that it's going to return.

This book will give you some simple strategies to deal with that fear and to get back your life.

CONTENTS

Hello and welcome

You've probably bought this book because you have come out the other side of cancer treatment. Maybe you're still battling it, and maybe you've been given the all clear but either way you'll be dealing with the very real fear the cancer might come back.

I am not a doctor or a psychologist. I'm just an ordinary person who has come out the other side of cancer treatment. Along the way I wrote a blog that helped a lot of people and they encouraged me to write some simple guides for people like you.

I know a bit about how you are feeling because this is where I live.

When I was 51 I had my first free mammogram. I spent the next few years having treatment for triple negative breast cancer (because why not get the rare, aggressive kind!).

Along the way I experienced chemotherapy, breast-conserving surgery, radiation, a one-year scan with some suspicious cells, and then another breast-conserving surgery followed by a double mastectomy when the cells proved to be active invasive cancer.

I also had a lump appear on my chest wall about one year after the mastectomy (thankfully benign) so I think it's fair to say I'm qualified to write about what it's like to be afraid of cancer coming back.

I met many people during my treatment and many more since it ended. A lot of us tell the same story. Ask us how we're feeling and, if we are honest, we'll tell you we are sometimes worried sick.

I find it interesting that so many of us use the phrase 'worried sick'. It's an accurate description. Too much worry can cause physical damage to our brains, our bodies and our immune systems. Sometimes cancer can leave us feeling helpless and hopeless.

But what if, instead of trying to push fear away, we faced it?

What if there was a way to harness our fear for our own benefit?

What if this fear could actually help us to live richer and more fulfilling lives?

I hope by the time you get to the end of this book you'll see there's a lot you can do with your fear and worry, and that it doesn't need to be a source of sickness. In fact, I hope to show you how to use it to improve your health.

I'm aware that often the advice other people give us is a bit like them handing us their reading glasses and being surprised when they don't improve our vision. These techniques worked for me, but how can you be sure they will work for you?
Well, firstly, because I've taught these skills to other people so I know they are quick to learn and easy to master. And secondly, because they are based on safe and well researched approaches for dealing with all kinds of fear and anxiety.

These techniques are based on Acceptance Commitment Therapy, or ACT, which is well supported by studies into everything from post-traumatic stress in the military to relationship counseling. It's been used by people all over the world for all kinds of anxiety, stress and grief. This stuff works.

I've woven in some gratitude and mindfulness. Many of these techniques have their origins in yoga and other Eastern practices but

I'm using them in a way that's not connected to any kind of religious belief. They're just simple ways to calm yourself and live your best life. You don't need to be any religion to use them and they won't be in any conflict with your faith if you hold one.

I'm also someone with a personal interest in the human mind and how it works. I enjoy reading about people who have rewired their brains after injury and articles about scientific discoveries regarding the human mind and body. Some of what I know about these subjects is in here too.

What I've come up with is a process for specifically dealing with the fears associated with cancer. You can certainly use these techniques to deal with any kind of fear. In fact, you can use them to deal with any kind of uncomfortable emotion, but because of my personal experience I'm particularly interested in helping people recovering from cancer, and helping the people that have helped them.

I use these techniques every day and I encourage you to do the same. They won't take you more than a few minutes and they don't require any special equipment.

I initially published this book on Kindle because it meant I could keep the cost down. Cancer treatment and the consequences of it mean that a lot of people struggle financially. I'm not trying to get rich (but a new computer would be nice). My main goal is to share what I know with other people because life should be fulfilling and fear can steal that from us. I got a lot of requests from cancer survivors for a real book. Many people don't have access to Kindle and I must admit I'm a fan of real books myself, so I decided to also release my work as a paperback.

I'm keeping this book simple. Most of us have some kind of brain fog following treatment. I've noticed a lot of self help books are padded out with repetition and case studies to justify a high cover price. This book gets straight to the point. I promise you I'll keep things easy to understand. There's no medical jargon or footnotes here.

This is a practical guide, not an academic work. You'll discover for yourself how effective these techniques are by doing them. That's not to say the book isn't well researched (it is). Just that I don't think you need me to prove that. Most of us know how to Google if we're that way inclined.

Because I'm teaching you something new there will be a bit of deliberate repetition. I hope I've struck a good balance between the need to remind you of something and the desire not to annoy you. Please know I won't repeat myself unless I'm emphasizing an important point (or my brain fog makes me forget I already mentioned it!).

My hope is that this book helps you to manage your fear and reclaim your life.

Don't read this book

I want to start off with a really important warning.

I've written this book for anyone dealing with the fear their cancer is returning but there are some people who shouldn't read it (or at least shouldn't read it until they've seen someone).

If you have any suspicion you might be clinically depressed or suicidal, you need to get professional help. It might be that a professional reassures you that you're just reasonably sad and upset by cancer but that's okay. Go anyway.

You should also get professional help if you are struggling with any form of unhealthy addiction. The techniques in this book are useful in recovery but you will progress much faster with professional help.

Please know this book is not a replacement for any kind of professional care. It's not an alternative to any kind of treatment and it's not about alternative treatments. It's just about practical ways to deal with the fear your cancer is coming back.

I strongly support the use of any professional that helps you recover, including mental health professionals. It was a session with a psychologist at the radiation clinic that first introduced me to these methods. You can certainly use this book if you're in treatment, but please discuss it with your therapist.

Do read this book

This book is for people who want to learn some practical strategies for dealing with the very normal and inevitable fear that cancer might come back from someone who has been there and done that.

You might call your fear by another name, like worry or anxiety, or you might express it as anger, frustration or withdrawing from life. These are all varieties of fear and these techniques will work for you too.

To get the most out of this book, I would recommend that when you come to each activity you **spend a bit of time practicing it before moving on**. Some of them seem very easy but turning them into regular habits takes time and practice (and you really need to make them regular habits to do any good).

Please keep an open mind and, even if you think something sounds pointless or a bit stupid, give it a try. The only thing you'll lose is a bit of time – and, just possibly, the distress and anxiety that your fear of recurrence causes you.

The methods in this book have been used by thousands of people all over the world with great results. I didn't make them up or invent them. I've just tried to put them into a format specific to people in our situation – those of us recovering from cancer. I've included some information on my own experiences with fear, and with how these techniques have helped me.

The feedback from my blog helped me to understand that sharing our stories is often the most powerful way we can help each other. That's why, when it's appropriate, I'll share a bit of a story with you. Some are mine and some have been generously donated.

If you're short on time, I promise that the activities I'm going to teach you will free up a lot of extra time. At the moment you spend it worrying, and worrying about worrying, and worrying about worrying about worrying. Or perhaps you spend it trying to escape your fear, only to find it follows you.

Even if you're a very busy person who thinks you don't have a spare minute, these techniques should give you more time to do the things you value.

If someone you love has cancer

Carers, partners, friends, parents and children of those who have cancer, or with loved ones recovering from cancer, will also find this book useful.

The activities are written for people who have had cancer but all of them are easily adapted to your situation. Your fear is just as real and just as potentially damaging to your health.

You'll probably easily relate to the situations and examples in this book. The experience of cancer treatment is different for everyone but there are some common threads. Fear is one of them.

I think your situation is often complicated by your wish to stay strong for the person you love. It can mean that your own fear, sadness, frustration and grief get pushed down.

It's important to process these feelings so that you can also return to living a fulfilling life, or can make the most of the time you have left while you continue to deal with someone you love having cancer.

Why we get frightened

There's a difference between knowing something and really understanding it. I've always known life was going to end eventually. Everyone dies. I worked as a police officer and saw a lot of death.

So why did the limits on my own mortality come as such a shock to me? Why, when I was told I had cancer, did my brain suddenly go into panic mode?

My father developed cancer in his fifties and, at the back of my mind, there had always been a concern for an inherited risk. But still. When I actually got the news, it was a terrible shock.

Everyone who has ever received a cancer diagnosis feels this. I'm sure you felt it too. When something becomes personal it suddenly becomes frighteningly real. It turns out when we imagine something happening to our future selves, like dying, we use the same part of our brain that we use to think about other people.

When we get a diagnosis or are in actual danger, we use the part of our brain that we use when we think about ourselves. Thinking about the death of some future version of us is very different to facing the present risk of our own death.

And so a diagnosis is very frightening. It's usually one of the biggest shocks of our life.

Then we calm ourselves down a bit, start treatment and come out the other side of it. We're not dead. We're almost certainly not the person we were before the cancer, but we're alive! For a little while we wobble a bit as we try to get back to normal.

At some point it occurs to us that we can never go back to a time when we were blissfully ignorant. Most of us spent our time before cancer living as if we were immortal, not really understanding how impermanent we were. We are wiser.

Over time, the stress of treatment recedes. Life gets back into a day-to-day routine and, for the most part, we forget about death and cancer and dying.

And then we don't.

Out of nowhere that icy hand grabs us at the pit of our belly. What if the cancer comes back? What if the cancer IS back? For some people, this fear can be overwhelming. For others, it's an occasional but still unwelcome intrusion. But why does it happen at all? Why can't we just get on with our lives?

Here's the first thing to understand about this fear: it's completely normal. **That fear is your mind trying to keep you safe.**

Our ancestors survived because of our ability to fear, and to use our imagination to consider the possible consequences of anything we chose to do. Movement outside the cave might be wind, but it might be a predator. Something sliding past our leg in the water might be seaweed, or it might be a sea snake. The churn in our guts after eating might be indigestion, or we might be poisoned.

Fear sets off a cascade of reactions inside our body that prime it for responding. Our heartbeat goes up and our ability to experience pain goes down. Our vision and hearing become sharper but our capacity for reasoned, logical thought suffers. Adrenaline is followed by cortisol as our body prepares for attack. Our physical performance improves so we can run or fight if we need to.

It's commonly known as the fight or flight response and most people are aware of the chemical cascade, but not so familiar with the imaginative side of this equation. In addition to physical changes, our minds also have the ability to store information about threats and to recognise the early warning signs when they happen again.

Because we have such great imaginations, our minds will not only send us a warning in closely similar situations, but in any situation where our brain recognises some similar element. This can be problematic.

It's why the food that made you nauseated at a party when you were a child will probably still make you queasy. It's why a single dog bite can make you fear all dogs, or a car accident can make you an anxious passenger.

We can also use our minds to create new scenarios involving similar risks and to develop strategies ahead of time. We can share stories with each other about threats we've survived or imagined so people can learn without having to face the same threats. This is why we might be afraid of a crocodile even though we don't live in an area where they exist. We can be anxious about eating in a foreign country because we've read warnings about food poisoning.

That's a lot of cognitive power dedicated to being fearful! All of this was once critical to our survival. Our mind is perfectly evolved to protect us.

So my first piece of advice is recognise that being frightened of the cancer coming back is normal and healthy. Your mind is trying to help you avoid something that was life threatening. It's employing the same strategies that our ancestors used to stay alive.

You are not crazy. You are not broken.

The trouble is this fear can become overwhelming. It can suck the joy out of life and leave us feeling distressed, angry, anxious or hopeless. It can leave us worried sick.

Fear gets a bad rap. A lot of people refer to it as a negative emotion, along with things like sadness and anger. But fear, like all our emotions, serves a purpose. It's a normal, healthy part of being human and once we understand it, we can use it to make our lives better. I'm going to teach you how.

First I'd like to deal with a few of strategies I see offered to cancer survivors time and time again, and why I don't think they are always very useful. Understanding why these methods may not have worked isn't just about helping you to understand why you might have tried and failed to deal with your fear in the past. Understanding the limitations of these traditional methods also helps you to appreciate some of the more important aspects of the methods I'm going to teach you.

Why what you've been trying hasn't been working

Most of the techniques I've seen for dealing with fear of recurrence fall into one of these categories:

Distraction: Keep yourself busy doing something else or deliberately think about something other than cancer.

Avoidance: Stay away from anything that reminds you of cancer and when you catch yourself thinking about it, shift your attention to something else.

Re-scripting: Listening to our self-talk and then rewriting it in a way that is supposed to be more functional or reasonable.

All these methods work well for some people some of the time. There's nothing wrong with them. The difficulty is they don't work for everyone, and don't work consistently. Let's have a look at why.

The downward spiral of distraction

Just about everything I've read about dealing with fear of recurrence recommends distraction as a strategy. We're told to go for a walk, watch a movie, play with the dog or bury our attention in a new hobby.

Some people distract themselves with healthy activities and others use food or drugs. Some people take dangerous physical risks to try and conquer their fears. Distraction is a 'flight' response to our fear.

All forms of distraction will work some of the time and there are some particular types of distraction that are really useful (more on that later) but for the most part, distraction isn't a reliable strategy. Some of us get caught in a downward spiral of distraction. See if this seems familiar to you:

You're facing the fear that your cancer will come back and so you try to distract yourself. You go for a walk, watch some television, maybe phone a friend. If you're like most people, the fear comes with you.

You find yourself experiencing a cycle: a little bit of distraction followed by a little bit of fear. You notice the distraction isn't working. This makes you even more anxious. You don't want to be fearful and now you're anxious about being fearful.

You stick with distraction and perhaps even change activities in the hope of stopping yourself from being frightened. It doesn't work. Or it works just a little bit and then it doesn't work. Pushing your fear away is like trying to hold it at arms length. It takes strength and effort and it makes your arm tired. Sooner or later you need to stop trying to push that fear away and then it's right back in your face again. So you have another go at trying to push the fear away.

This is a bit like trying to hold your fear above your head or behind your back while you do something with your free hand, but you know you're still going to get tired. You're aware of the tension in your body as you try not to feel your fear.

Now you notice the activity you're using to distract yourself is not a source of pleasure. Using it as a distraction has sucked the joy from it. It feels just like doing it with one hand while you use the other hand to push away the fear. You can't give the activity in front of you your full attention because you need to make sure you keep that fear at arm's length.

You notice that even though you're trying really hard to distract yourself, the fear keeps creeping back into everything you do. Sometimes you get short bursts of time when you stop thinking about the fear, and then you notice you're not thinking about the fear, which makes you think about the fear again.

You're frustrated. You're anxious about being frustrated and fearful about being anxious. The thought occurs to you that feeling this way isn't good for your health and now you're really upset! What if the fear of cancer is actually contributing to the risk of cancer?

At this point your fear might escalate, or it might shift into one of the many emotions that grow out of fear. These include the evil twins, worry and anxiety. Both recruit the phrase 'what if' to amplify your fear. You might also find yourself feeling angry, frustrated or annoyed. These emotions are a reaction to feeling out of control and fear is their foundation.

Does any of this sound familiar?

Most of us find distraction somewhat useful some of the time. You might be one of those lucky people that can just switch off, but for most of us, distraction is not an effective way to respond to fear.

Distraction is a bit like trying to pat your head and rub your belly at the same time. With practice, you can do it, but it's not going to become easy or fun. You might develop some pride in your ability to do two things at once. That's understandable. But you're still caught in a slow, downward spiral.

Here's why I think distraction doesn't work for most people; Remember what I said about your mind trying to keep you safe? Distraction means you're not listening. Your mind is sending you an important message about staying alive and you're ignoring it. What does your mind do? **It gets louder!**

We've evolved to feel fear and to pay attention to it. When we try to use distraction to avoid our fear, it's only reasonable our very clever brain will keep ramping up the fear factor to get out attention. After all, it's the reason our ancestors survived. Remember, your fears are not irrational.

You have had one of the biggest frights of your life. It was not imaginary. It was real. You've had several more frights along the way, probably involving test results, medical procedures and even the unexpected reactions of people. You have had a really, really big fright! Your highly evolved brain wants to stop you from ever being that frightened again. It wants to make sure you never put your precious life in that much danger again. You've correctly identified a major risk to your survival and your mind wants you to pay attention.

Instead of helping you to deal with your fear of recurrence, distraction does exactly what it has always done. It momentarily takes your mind off something. But your mind doesn't want to forget about cancer. Your mind wants to warn you. So eventually that fear is back up in your face.

Many people describe this as feeling like they are stuck. They get periods of time when things seem almost back to normal and then the fear sneaks up on them, or ambushes them when they're not expecting it. The methods I'm going to teach you will help you to overcome this pattern.

Please take some time to think about the extent to which you've used distraction to deal with your fears. How has that worked for you? Is it a reliable way to deal with worry or do you find yourself cycling back through fear again?

There's nothing wrong with using distraction if you've found it effective. It's just that most people don't. I'll teach you a better way of dealing with your fears so you can return to the activities you enjoy for their own sake, and not as an escape for your mind's legitimate concerns for your safety.

The other common strategy I see recommended is avoidance. Sadly, it's not reliable either.

Why we should avoid avoidance

Have you ever avoided something because you thought it would be unpleasant, or just because you didn't feel like doing it? You cancel out from a party at the last minute because you'd rather stay home and watch a movie. You stay away from the meal room at work because someone you find irritating regularly eats lunch there. These are normal ways to avoid things you find unpleasant.

Many people recovering from cancer think avoidance is a good way to reduce their fear. They have a mental list of the things that frighten them and they work hard to avoid anything on the list. Some people call these 'triggers'.

These people cope by avoiding the people and the places that remind them of their treatment or of cancer generally. They sometimes have just a few triggers, but may have many. They can usually give you a recitation of the things they seek to avoid. It's like their mental 'not-to-do' list.

Avoiding situations and people we find unpleasant can be a great way to reduce the stress and conflict in our lives, until it starts to do the opposite. Sometimes, in order to avoid triggers, we miss out on things we enjoy. Sometimes we just make our lives unnecessarily complicated.

Let me use a personal example to explain.

Many years ago I worked as a police officer. I lived in the same area where I worked. In the course of a shift I might get called to a death, a violent family argument, a robbery or something much more mundane. Every so often there was something particularly horrific to deal with. I found walking past the location where it had happened would bring back vivid memories. It seemed the best thing to do was to avoid those locations.

Over time it became more and more difficult to walk home. I would divert several blocks from the shortest direct route. It was impossible for me to get to and from work without going past one of these locations. It was about then that it finally occurred to me that avoidance might not be the best way to deal with things.

I noticed my journey taking me much longer than necessary, and it always involved me recalling a series of awful events. So the irony was that something I had done to avoid awful memories was actually reinforcing them. I couldn't make the trip without cataloguing the horrors.

Back then, police received very little in the way of counseling or support and no training at all in dealing with the distress that was a normal part of the job. Stress, fear and anxiety were seen as weaknesses to be overcome, or denied.

You can imagine my relief many years later when I discovered methods for dealing with my fears without avoiding them. I'm going to teach you those same methods.

I notice each October there's lots of advice for breast cancer survivors about how to get through a month of pink signs, displays, events, products and appeals. It might be a great month for raising money and awareness but many survivors find it hard going. Some actively try to avoid the pinkness. Some even give up wearing pink.

I've seen discussion in the forum of one very reputable cancer charity suggesting October might be a good month to stay home as often as possible. There was a lot of support for this idea.

Just like my journey to and from work all those years ago, these people are living lives that have been made more and more inconvenient by their avoidance.

We have good reasons to be fearful. It's not as if we're worrying because we decided it was a great strategy or a really useful thing to do. When people tell me not to worry I wonder if they've ever tried not worrying about something that really was a genuine risk to their life.

Trying not to worry is just another form of avoidance. It doesn't usually work.

There's a lot of advice out there recommending various forms of avoidance. I've even seen programs that get you to list every single thing you think will trigger your fear of recurrence. You then develop action plans for each one. How exhausting!

Here's the big problem with avoidance: in order to avoid your triggers, you need to be constantly aware of them, and of course, you'll now need to be constantly on the lookout for them so you can implement your action plan. So avoidance can actually require you to spend **more time and attention** on the things that frighten you. No wonder it doesn't work very well.

If you've tried avoidance as a strategy, you have probably also found that in spite of your advance planning, your triggers ambush you when you least expect it. No matter how carefully you plan, there's always something unexpected, and now you're stuck. If avoidance was your only strategy, what will you do when you can't avoid your fear?

There are also some triggers you just can't (or shouldn't) avoid. Your regular check-ups, surgery or treatment – and lots of other predictable circumstances – are bound to set you off, but how would you avoid these? And imagine the risks to your health if you do. Sadly, I have known people who stopped having their regular check-ups because of the distress they caused. This is the dark side of avoidance. Instead of helping us to live better lives, it might actually endanger our survival.

Please take some time to think about how you've been living your life so far and to what extent you've been avoiding certain situations or people. As I said, it's fine to make a decision about not having someone in your life, or not doing something you don't enjoy, but if you're avoiding something because you're frightened of the extent to which it will frighten you, then that's not healthy.

I read some research recently into Post Traumatic Stress Disorder (PTSD) in soldiers. This condition sees people in high stress jobs haunted by fear. They experience a range of awful symptoms that may include flashbacks, panic attacks, tension headaches, chest pains, irritable bowel syndrome, insomnia, mood disturbances and depression.

It's a wonder that all soldiers don't develop PTSD, but they don't. That's why this research was comparing different responses to traumatic situations. The researchers were interested in knowing if there was any difference in the psychology of the soldiers who developed PTSD and those who didn't. They discovered resilient soldiers were able to face disturbing situations, experience an appropriate emotional response (including fear, grief, disgust and horror) and also continue to do their job.

The soldiers who developed PTSD **avoided their emotional responses.** The soldiers who didn't develop PTSD were able to experience their emotions in real time, and to do their job anyway. This makes sense to me. Given what I now know about how my mind works, I know avoiding the things that frighten me is just ignoring a very important message from my mind. **So my mind gets louder.**

PTSD's psychological symptoms include depression, hyper-vigilance and vivid flashbacks of events. Physical symptoms range from headaches and chest pains to irritable bowel syndrome. Some people go on to develop fibromyalgia, a syndrome characterised by chronic muscle pain and cognitive impairment. All this, it seems, may be a consequence of avoiding a genuine emotional response to the event in real time.

Never doubt that fear can damage your health. PTSD is just one example of the serious consequences of untreated fear. It's as if the mind, having been initially ignored, hijacks the body to get our attention. Avoiding our emotions is potentially very bad for us.

Of course, avoidance can also be a good thing. Avoiding unhealthy choices in food, drink and even people can be extremely beneficial. Sometimes a decision to move someone dangerous out of our lives is the best choice but generally speaking, avoidance serves to make us even more frightened when we use it to avoid our fears.

It won't surprise you to learn my 20 years of policing ended with chronic PTSD. If only I'd known that trying to avoid what I thought were bad emotions was the least healthy thing I could do. I was the kind of person who tried to park my responses to the awful things I saw, thinking I could somehow get back to them later.

I would also try to avoid seeing upsetting things. A bundle on the side of the road might be a dead animal or a bag of rubbish, but I would avoid looking at it either way. It turns out I should have been facing my fears, acknowledging whatever emotions came up and accepting that these emotions were normal and healthy. I now know I should look directly at whatever is on the side of the road. If it is a dead animal I can acknowledge my sadness. What I have noticed is, more often than not, it's a bag of rubbish.

Just like distraction, avoidance has us ignoring a really important message about our safety. Our mind wants to remember what it was that frightened us, so we can actually avoid it in the future.

Refusing to process our emotional response leaves our mind unconvinced that we can keep ourselves safe.

If the threat to our safety was a savage animal, then avoiding that animal or running away from it would both be a great idea, but we cannot outrun our fear, or pretend it doesn't exist, or avoid it, any more than we can run away from cancer.

Tossing out the script on re-scripting

Most people are only aware of re-scripting strategies if they have been taught them by a psychologist or a therapist. There are also some people who have figured out methods for re-scripting on their own or learned them from parents or teachers. The goal is to pay attention to the messages your mind is sending you, to recognise categories of thinking that are 'dysfunctional' and to rewrite them. I'll give you an example:

Suppose you're getting ready for work and you spill coffee on your clothes. Because you needed to change, you miss your bus and when you get to work your boss is angry. Based on these events you now conclude that you are going to have a bad day. Re-scripting would teach you to identify this as dysfunctional thinking: Just because something goes wrong it doesn't mean that the rest of the day will be 'bad'. You learn, as an alternative, to acknowledge that the day was off to a bad start but that this is not predictive of anything.

The list of 'dysfunctional' thinking methods is a long one, and it includes 'catastrophising', which is probably better known as running a 'worst case scenario'. Re-scripting teaches you to recognise when you are doing this and to reasonably debate with yourself. It can be extremely useful for some people, but it has some serious limitations.

When my daughter was little she would become fearful before long car journeys. Thanks to someone carelessly sharing a news story with her, she was aware that sometimes people died in car accidents. Any time we talked about driving any distance she would ask, 'What if we're all killed in a car accident?' She was three. We would explain to her (in appropriate language for a three year old) that her thinking was dysfunctional (she was catastrophising).

We would remind her the actual risk of car accidents was small, that we were careful drivers and that we had made thousands of similar journeys without ever having an accident. We attempted to give her a new script.

Sounds like reasonable and caring parenting, doesn't it? She would usually calm down enough to make the journey, but I noticed she was always greatly relieved when we reached our destination. Over time, and many journeys, she became genuinely calm, but it took her own experience to change her emotional state, not our attempts at getting her to think differently.

I believe my daughter's situation is a good analogy for what happens when we try to reason with ourselves. Our fear comes from a primitive part of our brain. All animals have it. It's the reason so many of us experience a fear of snakes, spiders, heights or water. We're hard-wired for it. When you reason with yourself you use the evolved part of your mind, the part that relies upon language and reason. You **can** calm this part of your mind down by being rational, but the primitive part of your brain stays frightened. It's a bit like putting a fearful child in a car and making it very clear you don't believe they should be frightened. You will have an impact on their behaviour, but only experience will really shift their fear.

When we're dealing with irrational fears, this method has merit. The rational mind can override the primitive mind long enough for experience to kick in. A common example is teaching people to overcome their fear of spiders. The person is slowly exposed to increasing levels of contact with spiders while they repeat phrases to themselves about being safe. Over time the primitive brain stops responding with a fight or flight response.

So these methods are definitely useful for irrational fears.

The trouble is our fears concerning cancer are not usually irrational. Our health is genuinely at risk. In most cases there is a real possibility the cancer will kill us, or that it may metastasise and kill us in the future. Telling ourselves to be realistic about the risks just isn't going to help.

It's also worth mentioning a common response to fearful situations that's closely aligned to re-scripting. I think of this one as the 'inner parent', because it sounds so much like the way I used to talk to my three-year-old about car journeys. It sounds a bit like this:

There's no point being frightened about your surgery because you just have to have it. The doctor has performed this surgery hundreds of times and the risks are small. This is an excellent hospital with very good staff and your fears are not doing you any good.

I think this is really a tricky form of distraction. It sounds like you're being present and mindful but you're really trying to talk yourself out of being frightened. What you really need is permission to be frightened, and the ability to express that fear honestly. You also need some tools to help you keep that fear proportionate to the circumstances, so it doesn't overwhelm you.

The differences between the methods I'm teaching you and re-scripting are subtle, but they are also important. Everything starts with recognising your fear is normal and appropriate. It's not a naughty child in need of discipline, but a frightened child in need of a hug.

You need the tools to safely express your fear and the language to do it. You need the skills to accept your fear without it overwhelming you. Trying to convince yourself that you are not frightened when you really are might actually make you very sick.

Time for action

So let's get started. So far I have given you some background into why we get frightened and into why avoidance, distraction and beating ourselves up are not very useful. I've explained why re-scripting can feel like hard work and what happens when we try to use logic to convince ourselves not to be frightened. I wanted to start with all of these strategies, because most people rely upon one or a combination of them. Some of them will work some of the time for some people, but there is a better way.

I hope I have also explained **why** these approaches don't work reliably. Our minds are perfectly designed to protect us, to record frightening events and to use those memories to keep us safe. Most of the strategies we try to avoid our fear of cancer require us to ignore the very important message our mind is sending.

I used to treat fear as a symptom that needed a cure. I believed it was a 'negative emotion' and that, with the right kind of training, I could somehow learn not to feel it. This was not successful. In time I realised there are no 'negative' or 'bad' emotions.

In recent years there's been a boom in happiness. There have been books and programs and meditations on how to be happier, but the truth is that life is sometimes very difficult, painful and sad. All human emotions are part of what makes us human. We know this is true. When we look around us, we notice most people we know are happy some of the time, but nobody is happy all of the time.

Having an optimistic disposition is a worthy goal. There's evidence that being generally more optimistic is likely to result in a longer and healthier life, but even the most cheerful person is going to feel a whole range of emotions when confronted by cancer.

Hopefully by now you have learned that this is normal.

It might be the most frustrating thing anyone said to me following my diagnosis. 'Try to stay positive'. I would usually respond with 'I'm positive I have cancer!' (My apologies if you are one of the people I said this to, but please know I was frightened and ill. Even though I'm sure you meant well, telling me to try to stay positive is about as useful as telling me to attempt levitation!)

'Positive thinking' techniques have merit, but they are useless in the face of fear.

Shortly after I was diagnosed, someone sent me a list of affirmations to say every day. It included things like 'every day my body heals itself' and 'I am brave and joyful'. I don't take anything away from people who find this sort of thing useful (and once again, I appreciate the intention) but I seriously doubt the benefits of this approach. How does this let my frightened mind know that I've paid attention? There's a bit of usefulness to these approaches because at least we are being present and mindful but ultimately we're still ignoring our real and legitimate fear.

Please be reassured I will not be insisting on false cheerfulness or relentless positivity. You will not be reciting affirmations or sorting your emotions into 'negative' and 'positive' categories. Emotions are not good or bad. They are just emotions. It's okay to be sad. It's okay to be angry and frustrated and frightened. It's more than okay. It's normal, and human and part of what makes life fulfilling.

It was a huge relief to me to learn this. I spent a lot of time getting anxious about my 'negative' feelings and worried that they may have caused or contributed to my cancer. I found when I experienced the fear, pain, anger and distress that accompany cancer treatment, I would also double up by worrying about how this emotional response was impacting my health. It was exhausting.

It just makes sense to me that all my emotions serve a purpose. Nature is very efficient and rarely wastes energy. Our emotional responses are probably still playing catch-up from our lives as primitive humans, but that doesn't make them useless. It's true most of us are unlikely to be hiding from lions or hunting prey for dinner, but our emotional kaleidoscope is still our filter for interpreting all life's rich and wonderful experiences, even the scary ones.

How ironic that in giving up the quest to be happy all the time I am happier than I've ever been.

Hopefully the time you've spent reflecting on how you have usually dealt with fear has motivated you to keep going, if only to see if there is a better way. So you know something about what doesn't work. Let's move on to what does. Here are the five strategies I use every day to deal with the fear of cancer returning:

Take a moment

Face your fear

Acceptance: Hold hands with the monster

Be present and mindful

Find your focus

There's a chapter on each one coming up soon. Once you've mastered the techniques in each section you will have developed new skills for managing your fear.

After that I'm going to show you how your fear actually helps you to live a fulfilling life. This chapter will integrate everything you have learnt along the way by linking it to what really makes your life worth living.

Living your best life

I'm going to give you some easy activities to help you respond differently to your fear. Once you've mastered them, you can use them in any sequence at any time. Think of these strategies as a kind of tool kit. Once you learn what each tool does and how to use it, you can simply reach for it when you need it. Everything you're about to learn will harness the power of your mind. You are going to work with your natural desire to be well and safe rather than trying to ignore it.

During your experiences with cancer you've established some patterns of thinking and acting that have been used over and over again. When we do this, our minds recognise a pattern and lay down a neural pathway so we can easily find that path again. This ability is the reason we can learn to ride a bike as a child and never forget how to do it.

Our neural pathways are like a well-worn track. They can be very useful if the patterns they've recorded are beneficial, but not so great when they lead us into dark alleyways where we get beaten up by our fears. They have now become a one-track mind when it comes to responding to fear.

The good news is that neural pathways can be changed. If what you've been doing has left you increasingly frightened and frustrated, then I can show you how to fix this.

Remember, you can't learn to ride a bike without getting on a bike and you can't ride well without practice, so please give these activities a chance to work by actually **doing them**. Just like anything new, things might feel a bit wobbly at first but stick with it and you'll be rewarded with mastery of some very useful skills.

I've made sure this book has plenty of space for adding your own notes and comments. I'd like to encourage you to attack it with a highlighter pen, or to underline things or to tab useful pages if that helps you to learn these techniques.

Take a moment

Our minds are amazing story tellers. They can take us on a journey to imagine different futures or allow us to recall wonderful memories. They can help us to create stories out of nothing, including stories about mythical and magical things that only exist in our imaginations. We can use them to access the imaginations of other people by watching movies or reading books. Our minds really are incredible.

If only they weren't so good at horror stories.

Remember, our minds tell us scary stories to help us avoid danger. It's just possible some of our ancient ancestors were eternal optimists, but they probably got eaten the first time they wandered into a forest without considering the risks. They didn't survive long enough to pass on their DNA so we're the descendants of the scaredy cats.

Dealing with our fear means understanding the role that evolution has played in shaping our thinking. Our wonderful minds have an amazing ability to remember the things that have hurt us in the past and to warn us about how things might hurt us in the future. They don't frighten us for no reason.

When you're experiencing fear of recurrence, your mind is telling you a story. It's trying to get your attention, so it makes the story **really vivid** and **really loud**. Your mind knows that not getting cancer again is a really high priority for you and so it's going to regularly shock you with reminders. What a clever mind.

It's also going to set off a shock wave whenever anything reminds you of cancer. It might be some kind of campaign to raise awareness, or an anniversary associated with your treatment. It will definitely go haywire over news of anyone dying from cancer or any kind of physical symptom you detect in your own body.

I know how this feels. I've found myself unable to sleep in the middle of the night, or suddenly overcome with fear while I'm doing something pleasant. I've lain in a hospital bed and imagined all of the worst possible outcomes (including not waking up after surgery) and I've frantically waited for pathology results that gave me days of running terrifying scenarios through my mind.

I've had that experience of routinely checking my body and finding a suspicious lump, and then I've imagined all the consequences. I've anticipated the horrors of chemotherapy and the risks and indignities of radiation. Looking back, the one thing that strikes me is the reality was almost never as frightening as my imagination.

My fear used to overwhelm me because my mind is very good at getting my attention. I didn't just imagine the most likely risks, or the most common ones. I imagined the highly dangerous and very unusual ones as well.

If you're in treatment for cancer or out the other side of it you've almost certainly had this experience: Fear grips and sometimes overwhelms you. It might strike in response to a predictable event or it might sneak up on you and hit unexpectedly. It might wake you in the early hours of the morning or keep you from falling asleep at night.

If it's really bad you might even have physical symptoms like chest pain, gut pain or irritable bowel syndrome. You might get tension headaches or feel unable to eat. You might get flashbacks of things that happened during your treatment and try to swamp your feelings with food or alcohol.

Your problem is not your fear. Your problem is your reaction to it. You don't have to live like this. There is a better way.

I'm going to start you off with a really simple activity that you can learn in just a few minutes.

Most of us are familiar with the phrase 'taking a moment'. People might say they need a moment, they want a moment or they're taking a moment when they just need a short break to process something. I've called this first activity 'taking a moment' because that's all you're going to do.

It's also language you can use when you're feeling frightened. If you're around other people and your fear is threatening to overwhelm you, say, 'Excuse me, I just need to take a moment' and then do this exercise.

Full disclosure here. I know I called this book 'Free From Fear' but you're never going to be fearless. Only a fool has no fear at all. What you are going to learn is how to be free from the crippling effects of fear, how to make room for fear and how to leverage fear to live a better life.

Remember, you're not going to try to distract yourself, or push the fear away. You're not having a 'bad' emotion; you're just having an unhelpful reaction to it.

Activity: Taking a moment

Please try this activity now so you'll be able to get in a bit of practice for when you really need it. Read through all the way to the end and then come straight back and try it:

- If it's at all possible, find somewhere private to sit down. If you can't, just do this wherever you are. It will still help. Pull over if you're driving.

- **Close your eyes,** if that's not dangerous or uncomfortable for you, and tilt your chin down slightly.

- **Take a slow, deep breath in**. Pay attention to the way the air feels coming in through your nose. Feel your belly and your chest expand.

- Once you've taken a deep breath in, hold it for a moment and then gently let the air escape from your body. Don't try to force your breath out. Just **exhale fully**. Keep exhaling until you feel like your lungs are empty.

- Now place one hand on your chest and one hand on your belly. **Hold yourself kindly and gently,** as if you were a baby or a beloved pet. Wrap your arms around yourself if that feels better.

- Now take **five more breaths**. With each one count slowly as you inhale and count slowly as you exhale. Notice how your breath feels as it enters and leaves your body. Observe it without judgment, the way you might observe a breeze moving through the trees.

- Try to **make your exhale just a bit longer than your inhale**. You might like to use a phrase like 'I am breathing in', followed by 'and now I am going to breathe out all the way'. Say these phrases very slowly to yourself as you breathe. Keep noticing the air moving in and out of your body.

- While you're taking these five breaths, let whatever thoughts occur to you come and go in their own time.

- **Notice your thoughts but don't grab onto them**. Your thoughts might hang around or drift away. Both are fine. They are just thoughts. If you find your mind drifting, just gently move your attention back to your breathing.

- **Notice that your thoughts are just stories** that your mind is telling you. You don't need to think about whether they are true or untrue. Just notice that they exist. They are just thoughts.

- When you've taken your five breaths, open your eyes and look at where you are.

- **Notice** your hands and your body. Feel your clothing against your skin and your body against the chair or seat.

- **Notice** what's around you. The sights, the smells the sounds.

- **Notice** the temperature. The time of day. What is it about the place where you are that captures your attention?

How did you go?

Did you actually try the activity or did you just read through it and decide not to do it just now?

Please remember that reading about something and doing it are very different. As good as your imagination is, it's no substitute for an actual physical experience of something. You can read all about hang gliding and watch films about hang gliding and imagine hang gliding but none of that will compare to actually hang gliding. So if you didn't try this activity, please try it now. It's nowhere near as difficult or frightening as hang gliding.

If you avoided this task because you judged it as being a bit too 'new age' or soft then please know that it's been taught to men and women in the military and police forces around the world. If that doesn't help, then remember nobody is going to know you tried it (unless you tell them).

If it's easier for you, try recording this exercise on your phone so you can play it back to yourself when you need it. There are lots of recordings available online for similar short relaxation techniques but there is something very powerful about hearing instructions in your own voice.

Reviewing taking a moment

What do you think? Do you think this would be useful when that chill goes up your spine?

Hopefully you experienced a sense of anchoring yourself in the real world and of getting out of your scary imagination and back into your body. At the very least, you should have found this activity helped you notice the difference between what was in your mind and what was right in front of you.

I know for some people this activity seems almost too simple to be really effective but please try practicing it regularly each day and using it the next time you're feeling even a little bit anxious. One of the great things about this activity is how simple it is. It's also one of the problems; people read about it and dismiss it as just too simple to be effective.

Try practicing taking a moment once a day for the next week and see if you notice anything.

Most people find doing it regularly helps them to feel calmer and less anxious. You can have a big impact on your fear of recurrence just by adding this simple activity into your daily routine. You don't need to wait until you're frightened to try it.

I now practice taking a moment every morning before I get out of bed, and every night before I get ready for bed. I'll also use it throughout the day if something makes me fearful.

I have a friend who does this exercise every time she goes to the toilet (I'm not sure I want to pay that much attention to my surroundings when I'm in a toilet) and another who sets aside some time every afternoon to practice it in his garden. Choosing somewhere you already feel reasonably safe makes sense for your regular practice.

Think of this activity as a bit like brushing your teeth. It takes less time than a thorough tooth brushing and it will help your mind become calmer and more peaceful during the rest of the day. It is also a very effective way to improve your ability to get to sleep.

You will notice I haven't asked you to do anything about your fear. You're not trying to push it away or redefine it. You might find just stepping back from it allows it to float away, and you might find your fear keeps hanging around. Both are fine. The purpose of this activity is just to help you recognise where your thoughts end and you begin. It helps you understand the difference between you and the story your mind is telling you.

You are not your story.

I think the reason that taking a moment works so well is it helps us to remember our thoughts are not real. Our imagination is a wonderful thing but we don't need to fear it, even when it's trying to scare us. The stories are uncomfortable but harmless.

You might remember that I mentioned neural pathways earlier. Recent research into the way our brains work has discovered we lay down neural pathways, a bit like the way we can wear a track across a lawn by regularly walking over it. When we've been through a lengthy frightening experience, like cancer treatment, we've laid down some tracks that make us more fearful.

Taking a moment every day to intentionally calm yourself helps you to form new pathways that contribute to you feeling calmer all the time. Not only that, the pathways laid down during treatment can heal, just like the grass grows back if you stop using a worn track.

Let's break down the various components of taking a moment so you can understand how and why they work so well.

Closing your eyes separates you from the real world and allows you to look inward and to focus on what's happening in your mind.

Tilting your head down slightly helps to relax your shoulders and to release tension from your neck. This position is also naturally calming. There's new research into the impact our posture and body position have on our metabolism, particularly our endocrine system. This is not at all surprising to yoga practitioners.

Your first slow, deep breath gives you oxygen and calms your breathing. It's common, when we are frightened, for our breath to become rapid and shallow. This starves the brain of oxygen and this increases our panic. Taking one good, deep breath is instantly calming. Holding it for just a moment at the end of the inhale also helps you to slow down.

Holding yourself gently is a form of self-comforting. Most of us are good at comforting other people but we forget to extend this kindness to ourselves. Some people add a phrase like 'you're okay' or 'I love you' to this step. Many people find this quite emotional the first few times they try it because they realise how infrequently they have cared for themselves in this way. Using some kind of gesture really helps with self-comforting. Human beings respond to touch, even our own. You might prefer to hold your own hand or stroke your own forehead. Anything that helps you to feel comforted is fine.

Taking five deep breaths continues to improve your oxygen intake. Focusing on your breathing also gives your mind something to do. By giving your mind a single point of focus you're practicing the simplest form of meditation. You're not trying to exclude any of your other thoughts. The attention to your breathing just gives you an anchor point. Regardless of what's going on in your mind, your body continues to breathe in and out and you continue to exist in the real world.

Trying to make your exhale a bit longer than your inhale and taking a short pause between each helps you to avoid hyperventilation (where you get too much oxygen).

The two phases, I am breathing in and now I am breathing out all the way, are designed to help you achieve this. Say each syllable slowly – 'I.….am….brea.….thing.….in' – to a regular rhythm. If you would prefer, you can use counting. Both methods give your mind something to focus on, a bit like giving an overactive child a stack of blocks.

Noticing your thoughts is a way of letting your mind know you are paying attention. It also helps you to separate out what is imaginary from what is real. You're observing your thoughts, not trying to push them away. It's a bit like being a field researcher watching an interesting group of animals. You're interested in what's going on but you're not trying to change anything. This activity is calming and helps you to notice the difference between thoughts and reality.

Opening your eyes and noticing what's around you gives you a clear point of reference between what is inside your head and what is real. Some people add a phrase to this part of the exercise to emphasise the effect: 'Here are my hands and they are real. This chair is real. This room is real….' You can also just observe real things in the real world. This part of the exercise gets you out of the stories in your mind and back into the present. From here you can start to relate better to the real world.

I think this breakdown helps people to appreciate that practicing this technique is pretty simple, but there's actually a lot going on. This is why it works so well.

Banning the bully

I'd like to make a very important observation here about how we talk to ourselves. When you spend time observing your thoughts, please try not to punish yourself for having them. Many of us have learnt unhelpful ways of talking to ourselves, including calling ourselves stupid, foolish, dumb, ridiculous or worse.

Oh there's my fear of cancer again. I'm such an idiot. I know that worrying is a bloody waste of time. Shut up you fool!

These activities are not about bullying yourself or anyone else. They're about accepting the fact our mind is doing everything it can to help us. I think it's appropriate that self-bullying is often called 'beating yourself up' because that's usually what it feels like.

When we start to pay attention to our inner dialogue, many of us realise we have fallen into speaking to ourselves in a way that we would never speak to another person. Sometimes this habit formed during our childhood, because parents or teachers spoke to us this way, but often it's just that we tend to be much harder on ourselves than we are on other people.

Please speak kindly to yourself. Most people respond to bullying with fear and resistance and your mind is likely to do the same. Ask yourself if there was ever a time when you responded well to someone else's bullying. Probably not.

I remember the first time my yoga teacher suggested we should practice non-violence with ourselves. I had always considered myself a kind and compassionate person, opposed to physical and verbal violence unless it was absolutely necessary (like when it's needed to arrest someone violent).

It was a shock to realise I had forgotten to treat myself as kindly as I would treat other people. It's a habit that's taken a long time to break and I still sometimes push my body too hard, or speak to myself too harshly, even after years of working on it. Fortunately I've also learned to be gentle with myself when I fail.

When you have been through cancer treatment, you have already endured enough. It's time to be kind to yourself. These exercises are not meant to leave you feeling bullied. You should feel calmer and safer. When you are learning to take a moment, please keep this in mind.

I would recommend putting this book aside for a week or two until taking a moment becomes a regular part of your day.

Keep a diary or a journal, if you like, and make a record of when you take a moment and how it feels. Some people find it useful to also keep a record of how often they feel fearful, and to score their fear on a scale of one to 10 (or one to five). Others find this kind of record keeping just makes them more prone to feeling fearful. See which works best for you.

How we usually respond to fear

Welcome back.

Hopefully you've now spent a week or two practicing the first activity and you can quickly and easily get out of your imagination by taking a moment when fear strikes. (And if not, remember, nothing is going to change just by reading about it. You have to actually do something for it to make a difference.)

When we're experiencing the big bouts of fear about cancer this strategy is very helpful for what I think of as **emotional first aid**. It helps us to reconnect to the real world and to acknowledge our fears.

You might be one of the lucky people who only needs to take a moment to deal with your fear of recurrence. You're probably someone who was taught to face your fears, and to process them, when you were a child.

For the rest of us, it's likely that you are already experiencing some improvements. You're probably finding this technique helps you to feel a bit calmer, but, as I said, it is only first aid. To effectively deal with fear of recurrence most of us need a bit more. Fortunately it is possible to learn some new ways of dealing with fear that help us to become more resilient and to deal effectively with it.

I want to expand a little on the previous information about fear, because we need to understand it if we're going to face it. I'm also hoping you've had a couple of weeks away from this book practicing taking a moment so you'll appreciate the revision. (This might be the bit where you sometimes think I'm repeating myself. I am.)

Three ways to get frightened

The most common responses to fear fall into three broad categories:

We try to **run from our fear**. These strategies include trying to distract ourselves, trying to avoid anything that reminds us of our fear, trying to just ignore our fear or trying to pretend we are not frightened. We now know all these strategies just convince our mind we are not paying attention to something really important. They might work for a while and then they won't.

We **hang on to our fear really tightly**. These strategies include going over and over our fears, searching for information that builds on our fears (like stories about other people with cancer), getting together with other frightened people and scaring each other (online or in real life) and feeling like our fears are always with us. Worrying this way makes us feel progressively worse. Large portions of our day are dedicated to feeling terrified. Eventually this can get so bad that we are frozen by fear.

We try to **swamp our fear**. These strategies include eating more, drinking more or taking other substances to try and manage our fear. They also include bullying ourselves for being frightened. Not only don't these strategies work very well, many of them actually increase our risk of cancer. This type of behaviour is counter-productive and self-destructive.

Some people use one strategy predominantly and others move between them. You might have different coping strategies for different types of circumstances. All these coping strategies will work some of the time.

As I mentioned before, my strong advice is to get professional help if you're dealing with serious depression or any form of addiction.

You can still use all the techniques in this book safely but suicidal tendencies, overeating, substance abuse and alcohol problems are serious and you're probably going to see much faster progress with the help of a qualified person. Cancer teaches us that time is precious so the sooner you can get help, the better.

For every other response to fear, it's worth giving some thought to what is actually going on with your mind. Remember, it's trying to keep you safe.

I find it interesting that the language around fear often refers to being bound up or knotted in some way. We talk about the grip of fear, of being tied in knots, of being strangled or choked by fear. Most of us have a physical reaction to fear in some part of our body and there's often a correlation with our language.

People who hold tension in their neck and shoulders will refer to something as 'a pain in the neck' and people who experience digestive problems say something makes them 'sick to the stomach'. It's likely that this is our mind's way of communicating to us and getting us to notice our physical symptoms. We're not causing this physical pain. We're reporting it. (Just to be on the safe side, I'd recommend not calling anything a 'pain in the arse'!)

Dealing effectively with fear is about recognising the physical and emotional reactions in our bodies and using simple methods to manage them. If you're prone to avoidance or distraction then what you're doing is essentially trying to run away from yourself. You've tried to externalise your fear so you can escape it. But your fear is in your mind. You can't outrun it.

If you're prone to worrying then your fear has become all-consuming. It's possible you used to try distraction or avoidance as strategies (and possible that you sometimes still do) but because you haven't paid attention to your fear you clever, protective brain is now sounding a permanent alarm to get your attention.

This won't work

Sometimes we might try one of these common approaches for dealing with fear, with limited success:

Holding other people responsible for our circumstances

Comparing our own circumstances with others who are in a worse situation

Trying to pretend our fears aren't important and telling ourselves we're being silly

Reciting positive affirmations

Making 'to do' lists

Looking at the situation from a different perspective

These are really just variations on avoidance or distraction. That's why they don't work consistently. Some of them will work some of the time and there's nothing particularly wrong with any of them. It's just they will usually eventually leave you wondering why you are still so frightened.

So if distraction and avoidance are 'flight' responses to our fight or flight instinct, what does the 'fight' half of the equation look like? In the wild, this would have involved us using all that adrenaline and cortisol to kill or injure our attacker.

In the absence of an actual attacker, I think our fight response to fear sounds a bit like this:

Stop being such a baby

Well, after the lifestyle you've been leading, you deserve this

Of course you have cancer, you loser
You may as well just give up now

F@#ck you cancer! I'm not going to lose to you!

I blame my parents for this. They used to smoke around me.

When people talk about dealing with cancer it's often in very aggressive terms. We talk about fighting it, smashing it, destroying it. It's worth considering how useful this approach is to our health, particularly our mental health.

Your fight response might also involve doing something physically active to burn off the adrenaline and cortisol, which would be great if a lot of forms of physical activity didn't actually create adrenaline and cortisol!

You might want to take a moment to reflect on your own 'fight' responses to cancer. Did you have aggressive words or phrases that you used while you were in treatment? Are you still using them? How well is that working? Do you punish your own body when you feel frightened? What does that look like?

When the things that cause our fears are external then sometimes fighting them is appropriate. When they are internal, we are fighting with ourselves.

Just like avoidance and distraction, giving ourselves a good talking to will work some of the time. We'll berate ourselves into action or bully ourselves out of our own misery. This comes at a cost. Fights cause bruises, even the internal ones.

It's interesting to me that people with addiction problems often have very harsh self-talk. Having beaten themselves up, they then resort to drugs, alcohol or some other unhealthy behaviour to avoid the pain.

People who overeat rarely do so joyfully (and certainly don't have any concerns about their body image if they are joyful about it.). More usually, they feel ashamed and embarrassed by their failure to refrain from overeating and they berate themselves for not having 'stronger willpower' or 'more commitment'. Having done such a good job of making themselves feel truly awful, is it any surprise they resort to eating to make themselves feel momentarily better?

Recent research into addiction has focused on how isolating it is to have a low opinion of ourselves, and how authentic connection to other people who value us can make a significant difference. A rat in a cage with no company will overdose on heroin. The same rat put into a playful, joyful environment with other rats will choose not to take the drug.

When you've been through cancer treatment there are usually times when you've resorted to speaking to yourself like an angry parent, just to push yourself to endure something. You may even have had times when you were particularly harsh with yourself. These tactics can sometimes help us to face frightening things, but they are not useful or healthy in the long term and there are better ways to deal with the fear your cancer might come back.

Berating ourselves doesn't work for the same reasons that avoidance and distraction don't work. Our mind is not behaving badly and doesn't need to be disciplined. Our mind is trying to keep us safe, and is understandably upset when our response is to be harsh. When confronted with a fight response, our mind might retreat for a while but it will still **find ways to get louder** about the very real risks to our safety.

The big freeze

Freezing in the face of fear is not usually a recommended strategy but many people still respond in this way. They have a frightening thought and their mind gets caught in a loop. The same thought just repeats and repeats.

I can remember when I first found out I had cancer. My mind kept repeating the phrase 'I am going to die….' over and over and over again. I found it difficult to think of anything else. I couldn't eat or sleep and I even found it difficult to breathe. It was as if my mind was unable to do anything else but repeat this phrase. I cried. I wandered the garden. I cried some more. The phrase became the thought that was at the front of my mind, every second I was awake. It became a sound track to a movie, playing in the background no matter what I tried to do.

The good news about the big freeze is that your mind, generally speaking, doesn't get louder. The bad news is that it doesn't need to because it already has your completely undivided attention. When you're stuck in the big freeze your mind has found a way to hijack your life. You might have a great job, a wonderful home, a loving family, supportive friends and any range of rewarding interests and activities but suddenly all of that becomes background noise to your fear.

At the time of my diagnosis, my daughter was on an overseas holiday. We talked about waiting until she was home but realised, with social media and my inability to keep anything a secret, it was likely she would hear from someone else. My dear friend asked me an important question: if the situation was reversed and I was travelling when she received news like this, what would I want her to do?

I made life's hardest phone call.

We both cried. I tried to answer my daughter's questions and admitted we knew very little about anything and probably wouldn't for several weeks. I apologised for ruining her vacation and reassured her there was no benefit in her hurrying home. Nothing was going to happen in the next couple of weeks and I certainly wasn't about to die.

I told my daughter that although she'd just had some frightening news, it was worth comforting herself and seeking comfort from her partner, focusing on the present and what was right in front of her and enjoying her holiday to the best of her ability.

I recommended she not use future possibilities to scare herself because nothing had actually happened yet, apart from a diagnosis, and we really had no idea what was going to happen, but we did know that every single day was precious and worth living. (And still my mind played the sound track, 'you are going to die, you are going to die, you are going to die'.)

My daughter posted a message to Facebook. 'I know I'm supposed to say something deep and profound right now but all I can think of is f@#ck you cancer!' She didn't try to rationalise anything. She just expressed how she was feeling.

It was the metaphorical slap I needed. I realised the loop in my head was real, but it wasn't helpful. I also realised even though I had cancer, that didn't mean cancer was going to be the thing that killed me. I realised while the fear was certainly justified it wasn't particularly useful. I understood it was going to be completely unreasonable to expect myself to be fearless in the face of cancer. Cancer is very frightening. Only a fool wouldn't be afraid of it.

So there was no avoiding my fear, and no distraction likely to last for long. What could I do instead?

It occurred to me that my advice to my daughter was advice I should take. Comfort myself, focus on the present and what's right in front of me, enjoy life to the best of my ability and remember that each day is a precious opportunity. I needed to acknowledge my fear for what it was, a series of stories my mind was telling me to keep me safe.

I didn't stop being frightened. I did move my life to the forefront and allowed the fear to become the background music, like having a radio playing an annoying song. I could live my life and enjoy each day without it drawing too much of my focus.

I stopped getting stuck in a loop and I stopped making myself more and more distressed. I kept working on ways to deal with my fear and although I didn't know it at the time, cancer was going to give me a great deal of raw material over the next few years. I kept researching and reading and trying things for myself. I got help from a psychologist.

Eventually I discovered that the best way to deal with fear is to face it.

I sometimes think of my fear as being like one of those nets you see in old movies, the kind that activates when you step on it and hauls you up into a tree. That's how fear can feel. One minute I'm walking along enjoying my life and the next I'm all arms and legs and suspended above the ground.

When fear strikes it disconnects me from the people I care about. It drains the pleasure from things I enjoy. I used to struggle against my fear or just pretend it wasn't there. Neither worked. I now know I'm the one who set the net in the first place. The imaginary net is there to rescue me from the imaginary lion that's just around the corner in the imaginary jungle.

I now know the best way to deal with my fear is to spend some time examining the net, the jungle and the lion. I need to remind myself that all these things are imaginary and all of them serve a purpose.

Face your fear

Facing your fear is about recognising your mind is trying to grab your attention with scary stories. It's doing this to help you, but often it's not actually helpful.

I always wonder why people respond to my worrying by telling me not to worry, as if it somehow just hadn't occurred to me that my worrying wasn't doing me any good. I feel the same way about people who tell me things will probably be okay (particularly in circumstances where things are definitely not going to be okay).

If not worrying was as simple as just deciding not to worry, wouldn't I have already done it? Even if things really are most likely to be okay, would that mean all the other options weren't worth considering? And how does telling me not to worry help me to process my very legitimate and entirely reasonable worry? Comments like this usually wash over me because I appreciate people mean well. Sometimes they make me angry, which I suppose is actually a little bit useful because the anger tends to displace the worry!

I was greatly relieved to learn that the best way to deal with worry and fear is to acknowledge it, open myself up to it and allow my mind to tell me the scary story in all its glorious detail.

The only way I've found to effectively deal with fear is to apply these techniques. You've already learned to take a moment and now we're going to build on that.

If any of the following activities start to sound like a bully in your head, then please remember this: you are honoring your mind and its amazing ability to keep you safe. You are not trying to beat it into submission. If you know you're prone to this kind of behaviour you might like to review the section on banning the bully.

I'm going to get you to do a couple of short activities and then I'm going to teach you how to loosen the grip you have on your fear and the grip your fear has on you.

This first activity is very useful but you may find it unpleasant. I'm going to ask you to recall the day you received the news you had cancer. Remember, the past is just a series of stories in your head. This event is no longer real. Most people find this activity a bit uncomfortable but that's part of why it works. It's uncomfortable but it's also separate from who you are today, which is kind of the point..

Activity: Recalling your diagnosis

- Think back to the day you were told about your cancer diagnosis. Where were you? How did you feel? What did you think? Spend a few minutes really imagining it. What were you wearing? What time of year was it? Who else was with you? What else was in the room? How much detail can you recall?

- Notice what feelings this stirs up for you. You are bringing to mind a very unhappy memory.

- Now notice that even if this activity isn't pleasant, you are not feeling exactly the same way you did on the day you received your diagnosis. You might still be experiencing some anxiety and fear, but it will not be as intense as it was on the day it happened.

- Why not?

- What's different?

When I teach this to people face-to-face, they usually say something like: 'It's different because it's not actually happening. I'm just remembering it.'

Yes!

You noticed there's a difference between you and your thoughts.

Did you have a similar experience? Hopefully you noticed that even though the memory is not a pleasant one, you can recall it without feeling the same level of shock and distress. You can differentiate between where you are now and what's happening today from something you are imagining in your mind.

Here is you, in the real world, and over there is your memory. Hopefully you noticed it was possible to recall one of the most distressing days in your life without it feeling as distressing as it did when it happened. You could differentiate between the present version of you and the historical version of you. You could tell the difference between where your mind is right now and where it was back then.

Your memory is still there but the emotions you felt at the time aren't overwhelming you. They are not as intense as they were the first time you experienced them. You may have also noticed there were some things you can't remember.

We know very few people have perfect recall, so over time our recollection shifts and alters a little from the actual event. We also know some memories remain vivid while others fade.

My in-laws are wonderful people, and very dear to me, but they often disagree over the small details of the trips they've taken together. Was the boat blue or red? Did we see something in this country or that country? They are very well travelled and share lots of great memories but I'm always struck by the fact neither of them remembers the same events in quite the same way.

I used to see the same thing as a police officer. Attend a crime scene and speak to witnesses and you'll be astounded by the differences in their recollections of exactly the same event. Even simple questions about an offender's height or hair colour can result in surprisingly different responses.

It's a good reminder that my own memories are likely to be based on real events, but not completely accurate. It's not as if we have a movie camera in our head that keeps accurate real time records of everything we do. Our minds take notes. They keep information that is deemed useful or joyful and get better and better at not bothering with the less important information. We also reconstruct our memories over time, adding or deleting bits based on what we think is interesting, important or entertaining. This is normal. Arguments over what is 'true' are usually pointless.

I'm also aware any memory I have is going to be influenced by my own point of view. I'm seeing it through a filter of my own biases, beliefs and opinions just like everyone else. My husband was with me when I received my diagnosis but I am certain he remembers it differently. So does my doctor.

This helps me to differentiate between my thoughts and reality. What is real is what is factual and what actually exists right now. My thoughts are the stories my mind tells me. They might be based on real events but they are not real. **They are probably not even entirely accurate**.

Here's another activity for separating out our thoughts from the real world.

Activity: When life doesn't hand you lemons

This activity is a simple demonstration of the power of your imagination. It also demonstrates the impact our thoughts can have on our bodies.

- Imagine you've just picked a ripe, yellow lemon from a lush tree.

- You take the lemon inside and put it on a cutting board.

- You take a knife and cut the lemon open. You notice it's a particularly juicy lemon. The fresh, zesty scent of the lemon fills your nose.

- You cut a slice of the lemon and put it in your mouth. It's sharp and tangy.

- You cut another slice of lemon and suck all the juice from it. You feel the sting of the juice on your lips and the puckering inside your mouth as the tartness of the lemon moves across your tongue.

What did you notice? Most people experience the sensation of their mouth watering. Which is interesting, because **there is no lemon**. You know there is no lemon. And yet your body just responded as if there was a lemon. Once again you will have noticed the difference between you, the real person not eating lemons, and your thoughts about eating lemons.

This is how powerful our imagination can be. It's powerful enough to trigger physical responses in our bodies even when we know there is no real thing happening. This is also part of why dealing with strong emotions is so important. Constantly flooding our system with adrenaline and cortisol is not good for us, but if we don't learn effective ways to respond to our fear that's exactly what will keep happening.

Your mind has filed the memories about cancer under **very important, potentially life-saving information** because your mind is trying to make sure you stay alive. Unless you give those fears the attention they deserve, your mind will keep triggering physical responses in your body in exactly the same way imagining a lemon can trigger your salivary glands. Our minds are that powerful.

What I'm going to teach you now are some techniques for observing those memories in ways that make them much less frightening. These are all very simple and effective methods for facing your fears. They allow you to hold your fears gently, to observe them and to recognise them for what they are, your clever mind's attempt to keep you safe.

Activity: Noticing you're noticing

This is my favorite activity for facing your fear. All on its own it's been responsible for helping many people live more comfortably with fear of recurrence.

I recommend you read it through a few times before you practice it.

- Think about the last time you experienced the very real fear your cancer was returning. What did your mind tell you? Was it a single phrase? A story? A whole scenario?

- Really try to recall that fear as vividly as possible. Put yourself back into the middle of it.

- Notice where you can feel that fear in your body. Does it make your gut ache? Your neck stiffen? Your jaw clench?

- Instead of pushing the fear away, make room for it. Taking a moment. Imagine yourself expanding to make space for the fear.

- Listen to the thought. It probably sounds something like this: 'My cancer is back!' or 'My cancer is going to kill me!'

- Now add the phrase 'I am having the thought...' to your fear. Repeat this slowly and clearly to yourself. For example, **I'm having the thought my cancer is back.**

- Now add the phrase, 'I notice I'm having the thought...' to your fear. Repeat this slowly and clearly to yourself. For example, **I notice I'm having the thought my cancer is back.**

- Now build on this and notice the fact you are noticing your thoughts. Add the phrase, 'I notice I'm noticing I'm having the thought...' to whatever your fear is. Repeat this phrase slowly and clearly to yourself. For example, **I notice I'm noticing I'm having the thought my cancer is back.**

- Notice any difference in how your body is feeling. Notice the impact this exercise has on your mind and your fear.

How did you go? If you just read the activity but didn't actually try it, please go back and try it now. Even if you read it and didn't think it would help, I would encourage you to at least give it a go.

If you've only read through the activity without practicing it, there might be some part of your mind telling you something so simple couldn't possibly be any use, or that the activity is stupid or pointless.

This is not a helpful story.

You already know your mind is very good at telling you unhelpful stories. You need to give your mind the experience of actually trying the activity so you have the reality of it rather than what your mind imagines.

Most people report an experience something like this: at the beginning of the activity they feel anxious, maybe a bit frightened and certainly uncomfortable.

As they move through the activity, they notice that noticing gives them some separation between themselves and their thoughts. They feel the grip of their fear loosen, and their body becomes more relaxed.

Notice I haven't asked you to try and get rid of the fear.
Remember the lessons that distraction and avoidance taught us. If we try to push our fear away or distract our mind with something else, our wonderful mind will just get **louder.** This technique helps you to sit with your fear and see it for what it is. You can notice it without it sending you into a spiral of distress.

Can you notice the difference between you and your fear? Over here is you, the real, actual person. Over there in your imagination is your fear, but it's not you.

Here's another useful way to think of it. If you've ever seen a map of a city you know it can be a useful way to get from one place to the other, but the map is not the city. Our fears and our memories are like maps created by our mind to help us navigate life. But they are not life.

Once you've practiced this technique a few times, you can have it ready for the next time fear of recurrence grips you. It can be useful to start with taking a moment first, by holding yourself gently while taking a few deep breaths and paying attention to your immediate surroundings. Then add noticing you're noticing.

Once again you might be struck by how simple this activity is to learn and practice. No complexity. Just a few easy-to-remember phrases you add to your own thoughts.

I'm having the thought...

I notice I'm having the thought...

I notice I'm noticing I'm having the thought...

This activity works because it's the opposite of distraction and avoidance. You are paying very close attention to your fear. You're observing it like a doctor examining a patient. You are interested in what's going on but also apart from it.

This activity also works well for those who are overwhelmed by fear because it allows you to identify the difference between you and your thoughts. By calling your fear a thought and then noticing it, you let your mind know you've heard the warning and you're paying attention. This usually has the effect of at least taking the biting edge off your fear and you may find it immediately calming.

You have faced your fear. Your mind has responded by recognising you have paid attention to a genuine risk and it's not necessary to ramp up the volume. Your mind may simply let go of the fear in response to this exercise. It might also continue to grumble away for a little while, just to make sure it's got your attention. Both are fine.

It's probably occurred to you by now that the methods I'm teaching you are the direct opposite of most other strategies for dealing with fear.

When I first learnt this strategy it reminded me of the old fable about two people falling in a river. One swims against the current and drowns while the other simply floats with the current until they are carried to the shore. Part of the reason these activities are so easy to learn is because you are floating with the current.

There's one type of thought that deserves special attention. If you notice your thoughts and realise ending your life seems like a reasonable option, it's time to get professional help. It's worth remembering some medications can cause this frame of mind. So can the depression that often accompanies cancer.

Thoughts of suicide might be accompanied by sadness or anxiety, but they might also just seem like a good idea. You might calmly decide that ending your life is a reasonable thing to do. In either case, tell your doctor. This current is a very dangerous one and you should not float with it.

The next time you're experiencing fear of recurrence, try adding this simple activity to your practice for taking a moment and see what you think. It could be that this is all you need to separate out your fears from who you are. It could be that this particular exercise doesn't work well for you at all. Fear not! The next section gives you a mighty tool kit of activities for facing your fear. Surely one of them will be perfect for you.

More fear facing activities

So, to recap, you've already practiced taking a moment and you've added on the ability to face your fear by noticing you're noticing your thoughts. Hopefully, like many people before you, you've seen how these simple activities help you to be more comfortable with your fear.

This chapter will introduce you to lots of other activities you can use to face your fears. The reason for including so many different versions is simple. We all have different minds and imaginations. For example, some people find it easy to visualise things, like seeing a movie in their head, and others think more in words or feelings. Some people like to leverage their logical mind and others prefer things that are linked to physical sensations or emotions.

I struggled to meditate for many years because I couldn't see things clearly in my mind. I tend to imagine ideas and concepts rather than actually seeing pictures. When I discovered we don't all imagine things the same way, it was a great relief to me. I now meditate easily without worrying about seeing the visualisations. I have chosen meditation techniques that suit the way my mind works. You can do the same with facing your fear.

Please read through the following activities and try at least two of them. There's no risk involved in any of these activities. You can practice them in private and all they will take is a little time.

You don't need to try every activity. Consider this a menu. Pick out the ones you want to try. If something seems really unappealing, then skip it. It's likely it just doesn't suit the way your mind operates. You're very welcome to try them all if you wish and it can be (probably surprisingly) a lot of fun, but this is not a test. These are playful strategies for dealing with your fear and they should feel, well, at least a little bit playful! Everything new feels a bit odd at first. Feeling clumsy or awkward is normal. So is not getting it right the first time, and having another go.

You might also like to revisit this section of the book from time to time for a new activity. Sometimes a fear-facing activity works really well for a while and then our mind gets a bit bored. Trying something new will help if this happens.

Remember, not struggling with your fear or ignoring it or trying to push it away lets your mind know you're paying attention to the very useful warning it's trying to send you. That's why these methods are not only effective for dealing with your immediate fears but they also help to reduce your fears over time. Your mind recognises the fact you're paying attention. It's not necessary to scare you quite so frequently.

In time you'll experience fear much less often and at a greatly reduced intensity. This will allow you to spend more time focusing on things that matter to you.

We know how powerful our imagination can be. (It's been scaring us silly!) These activities use the power of your imagination in playful and effective ways to cope with your fear of recurrence.

Activity: The present

This one is all about being present and mindful. It's great at any time but also particularly good when you feel seriously overwhelmed. It's the easiest of all the activities because you don't need to imagine anything.

- Wherever you are and whatever you're doing, stop. Get somewhere quiet and comfortable if you can and practice taking a moment; breathe in, breathe out and hold yourself gently. Take another five or so breaths and focus on making the exhale a little longer than the inhale.

- Now start noticing your body and the things around you, but instead of doing this for a short time, keep it going. Examine everything around you in close detail, using as many of your senses as possible.

- Return to your day but with a focus on the world around you and your place in it. Notice how your body feels and where it comes into contact with the floor or your chair. Notice all the physical things around you.

- Take some time to really listen to the sounds you usually ignore. What is their source? Pay attention to the quality of the light, any breeze or air movement, the look and texture of the details around you.

- Notice the difference between you in your environment and the thoughts that are happening in your mind. When your mind tries to distract you, acknowledge the thought without trying to push it away. (You might like to say something like 'here is another thought' or you might just label it 'thought') and then refocus on the present.

You've probably noticed this one is really just an expanded version of the activity you practiced for taking a moment. It appeals to people who don't have a lot of time on their hands, or those who find creative visualisations uncomfortable or difficult.

Becoming aware of our immediate surroundings in this way helps us to differentiate between the present, real world and what's going on inside our minds.

If you've already been practicing taking a moment then using this activity when fear strikes, is probably your easiest option.

I generally use this one, or noticing I'm noticing, as a first port of call. If I'm still feeling too frightened to function well, I use one of the other activities to manage that fear.

Activity: Name your story

Most of us have a recurring theme to our fears. Our minds are wonderfully efficient. They will quickly sort through all the various scary stories they might use to get our attention and select the one with the greatest impact.

For example, during treatment I found myself getting very distressed about the possibility of never knowing my grandchildren. I also regularly returned to an almost obsessive fear of dying.

For this exercise I'd like you to think about your recurring stories. Is there something that comes up for you on a regular basis?

Now I'd like you to give that story a name. It might be 'the scary cancer story' or 'the doom and gloom story'. It might be more specific like 'the unborn grandchildren story'.

I think it helps if the name has a bit of wry humour about it but it's not necessary. Just give it a name.

When your fear strikes, use your breathing activity for taking a moment and then just name your story.

Ah yes. The dropping dead story.

That's all you need to do. Simple.

Giving recurring thoughts a name helps you recognise them for what they are; not real, not happening right now and just a story. It's also an effective shortcut for letting your mind know you're paying attention.

Remember, **please don't bully yourself**. Don't name the story in a dismissive or abusive way. Your inner voice should sound like a curious scientist making an observation.

Ah yes, the scary cancer story. I've seen this before.

Your inner voice should not sound like a dysfunctional parent.

So, you're telling yourself the scary cancer story again are you? What an idiot!

This type of self-talk is unhelpful and ineffective.

Take a bit of time to think about what you would call the story your mind keeps telling you about the cancer returning because you might like to use it in some of the other activities.

Activity: Thank your mind

This technique is really simple and adds a little piece to the last activity:

- The next time your mind tries to frighten you, just name the story and thank your mind for trying to keep you safe.

- You might like to try taking a moment first, by holding yourself gently, taking some deep breaths and noticing your surroundings.

- Now name your story and thank your mind. *Ah yes, there's the doom and gloom story again. Thank you mind.*

- If it helps, give your mind a name. This is a useful way to separate out your thoughts from who you are. *Thank you, Finnegan. I know you're trying to keep me safe.* (I have no explanation for why my mind is called 'Finnegan' except that it makes me smile.)

By calling it a story, and thanking your mind for trying to keep you safe, you've loosened your grip on your fear. You've acknowledged that while the fear isn't really useful, your mind is just trying to do the right thing.

It's a bit like a relative giving you an unwanted gift. You can just accept it graciously, appreciate the intention and then move on. No need to be rude.

And once again, please resist any temptation to beat yourself up for even having the thought. Your fears are not stupid. You are not stupid to have them.

Activity: Make it a movie

Many of us have had experiences during treatment that were shocking to us. The memories of those experiences can intrude into our lives in unwelcome ways. Sometimes we recall these so vividly they feel real. But they are not real.

You can use this activity for any kind of fear, including fear about the future, but I think it's particularly useful for flashbacks, where you vividly recall a particular event.

If you want to, you can use the story title you came up with in the previous exercise 'name your story'. You can also just come up with a completely new title for your blockbuster movie. It might be 'the hideous medical procedure' or 'the horrors of chemotherapy'.

This one really appeals to people with good visual memory but anyone can try it. See if it works for you.

- When fear strikes, take a moment. Recognise your fear is just a story your mind is telling you.

- Now imagine that story is a movie.

- You see the title of the movie up on a big screen. There's spooky music behind the title. It's written in big letters and there are scary images behind it. Your title might be something like 'The hideous return of cancer' or just the word 'CANCER' in big scary letters.

- Now play with the image. Take all the colour out of it. Switch the background music.

- Shrink the movie so it's a tiny box at the middle of the screen.

- Bring up the theatre lights and wash out the image.

- Mess with the focus. Turn the image upside down.

- Put silly backing music behind it. Add a few cartoon characters if you like.

- Use your imagination to play with the movie in any way you like.

This activity uses playfulness to disconnect from your fear.

Projecting your thoughts like a movie is a great way to remind yourself they have no more reality than an image on a piece of film. A movie might look real and a good one can really pull us in, but some part of us always knows it's just a movie.

Playing with the image reminds you that you don't need to be stuck with the same version of the movie. You own your thoughts and you're entitled to mess with them if you choose.

Activity: Sing it out

If movies in your head don't work for you, this activity might do the trick.

Turn your fear into a singalong:

- Reduce the story in your head to a single phrase or a short string of phrases. Here's a perfect example: **My cancer is back. I am so terrified!**

- Now sing it, either out loud or to yourself, to the tune of 'happy birthday'. If you don't like 'happy birthday' then try 'jingle bells', or 'twinkle twinkle little star' (it's best to choose something ridiculous or at least light hearted).

- Keep singing, either out loud or in your head, and notice what happens to your fear.

This activity is probably the one most people avoid because it seems a bit ridiculous but I promise you, it's worth a try.

I've sat opposite friends and actually sung their fears with them. It's surprisingly funny, not to mention the odd looks you get.

Probably best to avoid using it in waiting rooms and hospitals though. Sitting in a hospital singing 'My cancer is back' to the tune of 'happy birthday' might upset people. Of course you can always sing in your head.

You might also like to use a song that helps you to face your fear. My favourite is Gloria Gaynor's *I Will Survive*. You can insert your phrase as a replacement to the lyrics or blend it.

Alright now go. Walk out the door. Just turn around now, cause you're not welcome anymore....

Disco dance moves are optional.

I really love using '*My Boyfriend's Back*' because it's so ridiculous.

My cancer's back and there's going to be some trouble. Hey now, hey now, my cancer's back.....

There's a big difference between using music as a distraction to take your mind off your fear (which may work some of the time but is unlikely to work consistently) and using music to face your fear (which is likely to have lasting benefits). Think about the differences.

Activity: Leaves on a stream

I find this one particularly good when my mind starts throwing up lots of 'what if' scenarios. If you get yourself bound up in a similar pattern or even if you just keep repeating the same thought over and over, this activity can help.

- Imagine you are sitting beside a stream. As each thought occurs to you, take a good look at it, put it on a piece of paper or a leaf and float it on the water in front of you.

- As you place it on the water take a deep breath in and as you breathe out, think of the phrase 'letting go'.

- Some of those thoughts will get caught up in the current and whisked away. Others will float around for a while before they sink or drift. It's okay either way. Just let the thoughts come and keep floating them.

- Sometimes you'll get the same thought coming over and over. It's okay. Just put each one on the water and float it. Take a deep breath and as you breathe out think about letting go.

This activity has been a source of great comfort to me when I've been waiting to go into surgery, or waiting for some kind of treatment like chemotherapy or radiation therapy.

My mind starts imagining all kinds of possibilities, most of them seriously unpleasant. It's trying to prepare me for the worst – and I'm grateful for that – but it's not really helpful when I'm trying to be calm before a procedure or a treatment.

By taking each of my scary thoughts, paying attention to it and floating it on a leaf, I can let my mind know I'm listening, and that every single thought is being given its very own leaf to carry it away.

It also helps me to remember that my thoughts are just stories that my mind is telling me. I don't need to grip onto them or give them too much of my energy.

If you like, you can combine the activity for thanking you mind with this one. I often do. A scary thought occurs to me and I notice it, thank my mind for trying to keep me safe and then float it away on a leaf. Exhale.

Activity: Clouds in the sky

This one is very similar to leaves on a stream, but instead you use different images.

Think back to the activity about noticing your thoughts. There are two things here. First there are your thoughts and then there is the part of your mind that is noticing your thoughts. You might remember I've referred to a curious scientist or field researcher in previous sections.

The part of you that does the noticing is a kind of constant observer. All of us have one. It's that part of our mind that can step back from our emotions.

You might like to think of this part of you as your true self. For people who practice meditation or yoga this part of the mind is sometimes thought of as 'the higher self'. If you are a religious person you might like to think of this as your soul or your spirit, but you don't need to be religious to use this technique.

- Take a moment to hold yourself gently, breathe deeply and anchor yourself. Close your eyes if you wish.

- Imagine your mind is the clear blue sky. Vast and expansive.

- Imagine your thoughts are like clouds in that clear blue sky.

- As each scary thought occurs to you, imagine it is a cloud. Pay attention to the thought and imagine what type of cloud you will assign to it. Is it a small, fluffy cloud or a dark looming one?

- Allow the clouds to come and go. Some might hang around and some might drift off quickly.

- Notice that above the clouds is the sky. This is you. This part of you is constant and unchanging. It will still be here when the clouds have moved on.

- Notice that the clouds come and go but the sky is always there, even when it's completely hidden by clouds.

- Repeat the phrase 'I am the sky. My thoughts are the clouds' to yourself.

When fears threaten to overwhelm you, recall this image and remind yourself: 'I am the sky and my thoughts are the clouds'. Remember, your thoughts have no power to harm you. They are just ideas inside your head.

Notice how your thoughts and emotions change like the weather changes. Sometimes there are lots of clouds and sometimes only a few. Sometimes the clouds move away quickly and sometimes they hang around for a while, but sooner or later they move on.

This one is my alternative to leaves on a stream and also very effective for me when I am dealing with really acute fear.

I used it when I received the news my cancer had returned and I needed a mastectomy. It was a terrifying time. Reminding myself that I was the sky and my fear was the clouds got me through that. I could acknowledge my fear was very real and entirely justified. Also that it would eventually pass, just like bad weather.

I can now summon up this imagery quickly, just by saying 'I am the sky'. This immediately makes me calmer. Regular practice can give you that ability too.

Once again, you can add thanking your mind to this activity very easily if you find that is helpful.

Activity: A trip to the zoo

This activity draws on an actual memory most of us are familiar with, so I think it's one of the easiest. Trying to shrink movies or imagine clouds leaves some people cold and others feeling inadequate.

It's helpful to remember that not everyone is able to clearly visualise things. Some people think in words or impressions instead of pictures.

Using an actual memory can be a great way to harness the power of your mind to your advantage. See what you think of this one.

- Remember the last time you visited a zoo. Recall a time when you stood in front of a glass wall or a cage and looked at a dangerous wild animal inside it. You can choose any animal you like but make it something lethal, like a tiger or a crocodile.

- Try to make the memory as vivid as possible. Which zoo was this? Who was with you? What was the weather like? Can you remember what you wore?

- Now remember how you were feeling. You were very close to a seriously dangerous animal but you weren't frightened. Why not?

- You knew the animal was the other side of the glass. It was still a very dangerous and potentially lethal animal, but you knew you didn't need to be afraid of it because there was a barrier between you and the animal.

- Now name that animal 'fear of cancer'; fear of cancer the tiger; fear of cancer the crocodile. Whatever scary animal you choose, give it that name.

- Notice how you can look at your fear of cancer through the glass and not be afraid of it. Cancer is dangerous and potentially lethal but your fear of it is like a caged animal in a zoo. You are safe from it. There is a barrier between you and your fear.

I have a friend who didn't have a recent memory of going to a zoo who found this activity really appealing. He worked it the other way around. He headed off to the nearest zoo and sat outside the tiger's cage, calling it 'fear of cancer' for about half an hour. He tells me it was a great way to loosen his grip on his fear.

If activities that rely on imagination leave you cold, you might like to try a real trip to the zoo. Your memories or imaginings about the future are your scary thoughts. Just like the animal in the zoo, they are separated from the real you. They exist in the past or the future, behind the glass.

Activity: Expanding

If you're a person who is more likely to respond to feelings and emotions then this activity will probably appeal to you. Even though I'm a bit of a thinker this one is deeply useful to me, so don't abandon it just because you're more of a logical type.

- The next time you're feeling frightened, find somewhere quiet and comfortable to sit. Take a moment. Hold yourself gently and breathe deeply but hold back from opening your eyes for now.

- Turn your attention inwards and notice where you feel your fear. Is it in your gut? Your neck? All over your skin?

- What does it feel like? It might be a clenching or a stabbing type of feeling. It might feel like pressure on the outside of your body or like some kind of internal build-up that's trying to escape. We all have different experiences and there's no right or wrong way to feel, so just notice what your experience feels like.

- Find the edges of your fear. Where does it begin and end? Is it flooding the whole of your body or is it stronger in some parts than others?

- Tighten up against the fear. You can imagine this or you might actually like to clench your fists, pull your shoulders up to your ears or hug your arms around your body. (I find just pushing my arms in hard against my sides does it for me.)

- Now let go of that tension. Imagine you're expanding around that fear and making plenty of room for it. The fear is still there but now it's released from your tightening.

- Notice the fear is still there but you have made more room for it. Take a few more calming breaths.

- Now reconnect to your surroundings by opening your eyes and noticing.

This activity is the reason I encourage you to try things that don't initially appeal to you. I didn't think I would find this activity helpful but it's been a powerful strategy for relaxing my body.

I have noticed my fear isn't just a series of thoughts that happen in my mind. It's also a series of knots I hold in my body. This activity helps me to find those knots and loosen them. I've also noticed some people regularly feel fear in the same part of their body and others experience it different places at different times. Both are normal.

Activity: Computer games

If you enjoyed the movie *The Matrix*, then this might resonate with you. It also works well for people who enjoy computer games, and fans of science fiction, but anyone can try it.

- The next time you find yourself experiencing the fear of your cancer coming back, find somewhere quiet to sit. Take a few deep, calming breaths and close your eyes.

- Now imagine you are not actually in your own body but sitting in front of a computer screen playing a game. The person feeling frightened is just an avatar, a character in a game you are controlling.

- Imagine you can decide what this avatar feels and how it responds to the world around it. Imagine using the controls on your computer to help your avatar sit with their fear without feeling terrified.

I know this one is the direct opposite of taking a moment but it can be particularly helpful when you're feeling intensely frightened. It allows you to rise above the fear a to be a bit playful with it.

Although this one feels a bit like avoidance, it isn't. You're still dealing with your fear. You're just using your imagination to take a step back from it and to recognise it's a game your mind is playing.

Activity: Oh look! Actual activity!

If you're the kind of person who loves physical activity, this one will appeal to you. Even if you're a more sedentary kind of person it can be useful, and it might just give you the motivation to be more active.

- When fear strikes, use taking a moment.

- Acknowledge your fear and say to your mind, 'Let's take that fear for a walk.'

- Head off on a nice walk and pay attention to what is around you.

- Also pay attention to the fear in your mind but don't hold it too tightly. Imagine it's coming with you for a walk like a friendly dog.

- The dog might walk along with you for a while or it might wander off somewhere. Both are fine.

- Notice your fear and notice you can still enjoy your walk and everything around you.

You can substitute any sort of physical activity into this exercise. You might like to take your fear bike riding, or to a yoga class. You might decide to take your fear dancing or swimming. The whole point is to get active.

This technique shows your mind that you're paying attention by doing something healthy. You've heard the warning about cancer and now you're actively doing something to reduce your risk. You might even like to thank your mind for the motivation to become more active.

You can also substitute any kind of animal, or just imagine your fear as a thought in your head that you are taking for a walk.

The main thing to remember is that you're taking that fear with you and not trying to run away from it. That would be counterproductive. Your mind needs to know that you are paying attention to the very reasonable message it is sending you. If you run away it will follow you and, if it needs to, it will bite you on the leg to get your attention.

Activity: Put it on paper

This activity is great and, unlike the others, you don't need to be experiencing fear of recurrence to practice it. I tossed up about putting this activity first because it's so useful and powerful but it's also fairly complex so I've opted to use it as the grand finale for this section of the book. See what you think.

There's a practical aspect to this activity that really appeals to me. I know it makes perfect sense to use the mind, and our imagination, to deal with something that's in our mind, but what if our mind needs something more concrete?

Somehow, taking our fears out of our mind and putting them on paper, and then using that paper as an actual tool, is very powerful. Some people are creative and artistic. Some are better with words. You can adapt this activity to suit your own preferences. You'll also need to wear something with a back pocket to do this exercise.

- Take a piece of paper and put your fears on it.

- Use words or pictures and any kind of method you like. Nobody is going to see this, so please yourself with which methods you use and try not to judge the result. If you'd rather write your fears out as a list or a poem or a collection of words, that's great too. Just get them onto the paper.

- Take the piece of paper and hold it in front of your face, almost touching your nose. This is what it's like when you can't face your fears calmly. You can't see anything but your fears. Notice when your fears are here you can't do any of the things that matter to you. You can't engage with the

92

people who matter in your life, do any of the things you enjoy or even walk across the room.

- Take the paper away from your face and hold it out at arm's length. Really try to push that fear away. Notice how the world comes back into focus. You can hold your fears and still create some distance that allows you to appreciate everything you really care about, but you can't really do very much while you're trying to push your fears away.

- Now take your fears and rest them in your lap. Let go of them. You'll still be able to notice them and you can even look down and give them your attention, but now you're free to use your hands and your eyes and all your other senses. This is what it's like when you face your fears and just accept them for what they are.

- Fold up the paper and tuck it into your back pocket. Notice you haven't destroyed your fears. You still have them on your piece of paper.

- Reconnect to the world around you and notice three things you can see, three things you can hear, three things you can feel and three things you can touch. (You can add your sense of smell as well, if that's appropriate, but we often don't have three smells available to us without moving around).

- Find a way to carry your piece of paper with you, either in your wallet, pocket or bag. Take it with you and, when fear starts to come up, thank your mind and remind yourself you have already paid close attention to this story and that you have it on you.

- If your mind throws up something new you might like to get your paper out and add something to it, but only if you think that will help.

- If you really feel overwhelmed you might like to repeat the process of putting that paper up to your nose, out at arm's length, in your lap and then back in your pocket.

This activity involves a bit more work than the others but it's very effective.

Sometimes just the act of putting all our fears onto paper provides a surprising amount of relief from them. Of course, you probably now understand why. What better way to let your mind know that you're paying attention?

Practice builds ability

I'd recommend putting this book aside for a while so you can experiment with some of the activities for facing your fear. Remember, reading about them is very different to doing them. That's why I called them 'activities'. You need to act to make a difference.

Please keep in mind that an activity that didn't initially appeal to you might actually work really well when you try it. It's impossible to fail at this if you remember you are only learning, and all learning involves mistakes, setbacks and starting over.

You would never learn to juggle if you weren't prepared to drop whatever you were juggling. You would never learn to play music if you didn't make it safe to sound a wrong note.

Think back to when you were a baby and just starting to walk. You would stand up and fall down. You did this over and over again but you didn't beat yourself up for not being able to walk. Hopefully, like most of us, you also had loving and caring people around you to encourage you and help you to balance. It's time to provide that loving care and support to yourself, to be your own parent while you learn something new and challenging.

It's probably not helpful to try all of these in a short space of time. Maybe choose just one of them and try it for a few days before moving on to the next. There's no time frame for any of this. Some people take to facing their fear like ducks to water and some need a bit more swimming practice. Be gentle with yourself.

You've already been through so much and the last thing you need now is more stress and anxiety, so please approach these activities with a light heart. They are an opportunity to learn something that will make life much better but they are not meant to be difficult or stressful.

I've included a range of activities from very simple to more complex but that doesn't mean the complex ones are better. They're just different. If something simple works for you, that's great.

You might like to keep a diary or a journal of your experiments with facing your fear. It can be fun and useful to keep a record of your experiences. But you don't have to.

Facing my fears always reminds me of a cartoon I saw as a kid. A mouse managed to terrify a cat by standing in front of a torch and throwing a huge, scary shadow onto the wall. Our fears often do the same. They exaggerate to get our attention, but when we take the time to look closely at them, many turn out to be just a mouse with a torch.

Now you've faced your fear

How did you go? Did you try a couple of the activities? Did any really appeal to you? Did some of them seem a bit odd or silly? Did you try them anyway? (I hope so).

Different techniques work well for different people. That's why I've given you some choices. There's also nothing to stop you from coming up with your own activities. Just be careful to avoid anything that tries to abolish your fear.

You may have come across visualisations or activities that involve writing your fear on paper and burning it, or imagining that you've put it on a white board and then rubbing it out. I don't think these activities are helpful.

We now know that is because our fear is not something we need to run away from or abolish. When we try to stop our mind from keeping us safe it just pushes harder.

Using the activities in this book regularly will build your mental agility. Just like physical activity, the more you practice them the better you will get. You'll also start to develop some resilience. Your fear is going to keep happening but now you've got some simple and powerful ways for responding to it.

Hopefully by this stage of the book you're already practicing taking a moment on a regular basis and you've had some early experiences of facing your fear. You should already be noticing some benefits. These will keep improving with practice.

I now know I'm not going crazy and that when fear strikes I have a whole stash of activities I can use. I know that feeling fearful doesn't make me broken. It's just a normal part of being human.

I've also found these activities useful for other emotions. When I'm angry or frustrated or feeling anything else uncomfortable, I can quickly take a moment and then face that emotion. I can experience what my mind is telling me and respond to the emotion without feeling overwhelmed by it.

I still feel the full range of human emotions but I now react very differently to them. Accepting that emotions like anger and fear are actually protective has been such a huge shift for me.

I hope by now you have also had the experience of facing your fears and seeing them for what they really are. Fears are not a terrifying monster but a kind, if somewhat annoying friend.

Next I'm going to introduce you to the concept of acceptance.

Acceptance: Hold hands with the monster

It's difficult to find a lot of resources on acceptance. There's plenty on mindfulness and gratitude and being present (more on those later) but very little about the power of acceptance and why it can be so useful to us.

I think of acceptance as holding hands with the monster because it reminds me of those fairy tales where the hero manages to make friends with their enemy rather than killing it. (I always preferred those.)

You probably know the tale about the lion with the thorn in his paw that makes friends with the person who removes it. Often the 'enemy' in these stories winds up being a well-meaning beast that is just misunderstood.

It reminds me of what I've learned about my fear. I used to regard it as a monster that needed to be conquered. Now I understand my fear is uncomfortable, but it's not dangerous or negative if I know how to manage it.

I'm sure the reason the Disney song *Let It Go* from the movie *Frozen* was such a big hit had something to do with our ability to recognise the power of acceptance. It's the point in the movie where the main character accepts herself for who she is.

She's letting go of all of her attempts to please other people and facing all of her fears about her magical abilities. She's even a bit playful with it: 'The cold never bothered me anyway.'

Acceptance allows us let go of our desire to control the uncontrollable. As a police officer I used to see people battling with control all the time. They thought that somehow they were going to change and abusive partner, fix a suicidal teenager or conquer an addiction just by trying harder.

I think it's our egos that fool us into believing we have more control than we actually do. It can feel weak to surrender, but it might be exactly what we need to do to finally become strong. I think the best way to explain what I mean by acceptance is to get straight into an activity. See what you think of this one.

Activity: Let it be

For this exercise, I'm going to use a familiar experience for anyone who has been through cancer treatment. I want you to imagine you're attending an appointment with one of your medical team.

For most of us, these visits are a source of anxiety. Our fear will be worse if we've been using distraction to avoid thinking about cancer, because an appointment makes thinking about it inevitable and our minds take the opportunity to overload us with fear.

Even for those of us practiced at managing our fear, there's usually some trepidation about appointments. You're welcome to use any other event that reliably causes you anxiety if this one doesn't. It's just a suggestion.

You can also adapt this activity and use it when you are actually in a waiting room. It's really useful.

- Practice taking a moment. Get yourself calm and connect to your body and the space around you. You are safe.

- Imagine yourself walking into the waiting room for an appointment with one of your specialists. Notice the changes in your body as you start to experience fear, worry or anxiety.

- Use one of your 'facing your fear' activities and notice what happens to your fear. Remember, it's not going to magically vanish but you are going to be able to feel it, and still go through with the appointment.

- For example, I like to imagine my fear is a sharp rock in my belly. Instead of clenching around it (which would hurt) I expand the space and imagine it filling with flowers and plants. I create a garden for my fear. The sharp rock doesn't go away but I can be comfortable with it.

- Soothe yourself with any (or all) of these phrases:

  It is what it is.

  What will be will be.

  I accept this.

- Take a few more calming breaths and notice how you're feeling.

Reciting phrases like 'what doesn't kill me makes me stronger' are popular with some people but they are different to practicing acceptance. They get you to focus on the future rather than the present. If using this kind of phrase is effective for you, there's nothing wrong with that. If they don't work well for you it's probably because you're using them in an attempt to escape your fear rather than face it.

You can also use phrases like these:

Breathe into it.

Let it go.

Just let go.

I am right here right now.

This too shall pass.

Tomorrow is another day.

The last two of these are a bit contentious because they could be interpreted to be a shift in focus to the future. I prefer to couple them with another phrase that grounds them in the present. 'I am here, right now, going through this and this too shall pass.' 'I am here, today, experiencing this and tomorrow is another day.'

Both are a form of acceptance that helps to remind us everything is transient. You can accept what is happening right now and also remind yourself that it will stop.

My yoga teacher encourages us to 'be in the body you have today'. It's a great lesson in acceptance. I might have pain or physical restrictions today but who knows what my body will be like tomorrow, or next week, or next year.

You might also like to come up with your own phrase. The only requirement is that it anchors you in the present moment and helps you to accept what is happening.

You'll notice none of these phrases involve judging your circumstances as good or bad. Acceptance is about suspending judgment. It is what it is. You're also not judging your emotional response as good or bad, functional or dysfunctional. Whatever emotions come up for you are simply named and accepted.

Just like facing your fear, I believe acceptance is a way to reassure your mind that you are dealing with the situation at hand. This has a calming effect. Phrases like 'what doesn't kill me makes me stronger' might work for some people in the short term, but in the longer term you're still going to need to deal with that residual fear.

Not only that, but failing to process your genuine emotions in real time isn't good for you. Emotionally healthy people can describe what they are feeling, when they are feeling it. They get just as angry, terrified, frustrated, annoyed and worried as the rest of us. What makes them different is their ability to recognise the emotion and continue to function well, even while they are feeling it.

Acceptance can help you to develop your emotional resilience. Imagine if the next time someone cuts you off in traffic you recognise and name your anger or annoyance, accept that some people are just discourteous (it is what it is), and then let it go.

Acceptance doesn't avoid our various emotional states but it is very soothing. I find my ability to now say 'I am feeling really angry about that' rather than throwing the adult equivalent of a minor tantrum, has made life a lot more enjoyable (particularly for my husband!).

I have found adding these soothing phrases in those circumstances when my fear is really strong can make a big difference. My fight or flight response has my mind screaming '**do something!**' and these phrases help me to calm that monster.

I'm not fighting with myself. I'm not bullying myself by telling myself I'm stupid. I'm not using logic to convince myself to do something unpleasant. I'm just accepting it. This is very different to what my internal dialogue used to sound like. See if this is familiar:

'Look, there's no point being a baby. You know you're going to have to have this procedure so you might as well suck it up. Nobody wants

to hear about your problems. There are plenty of people worse off than you. Let's just get this over with...'

Or this?

'Okay, go to your happy place. Think about something pleasant, like the beach on a nice day, and just imagine being there. Don't look at the equipment. Just close your eyes and pretend to be somewhere else. Lalalalala.'

Now compare this:

'I am frightened. It is what it is. What will be will be. It's okay to be frightened. Who wouldn't be? But I can still be calm and frightened. I accept this.'

I have noticed once I accept my fear and breathe into it, I can usually spend the rest of my time enjoying the company of whoever is supporting me through whatever I'm about to face. My fear is still there, but it's well behaved.

The real challenge is to practice this the next time you're heading towards one of those situations that usually makes you anxious. Practice it beforehand so you know what you're going to do.

If it's possible, take someone with you and explain this technique beforehand, so they can support you.

I usually ask my husband to just hold my hand, or hug me, or chat with me about mundane things rather than giving me well-meant advice. He also understands that when I say I just need to calm myself down, I'm probably going to sit there with my eyes closed for little while. Having him next to me makes this feel safer.

If you're in a relationship then sharing these techniques with your partner is a good idea. As well as supporting you, they can also use them (having a partner with cancer can be stressful!). They will also be able to suggest activities when fear tries to overwhelm you.

It might earn you some strange looks when your partner suggests you 'take a moment', but I'm sure neither of you will mind.

I find holding hands with the monster (that's my fear, not my husband!) works particularly well when my fear appears in the early hours of the morning. I sometimes wonder what it is about the human brain that makes it want to wake us up with the cold horrors in the middle of a good night's sleep!

I now thank my mind for trying to keep me safe and use this activity to soothe myself. It is what it is. What will be will be. I accept this. I usually find I can get back to sleep relatively easily.

Acceptance exercises are also very useful if you're having trouble falling asleep. Try something like clenching and unclenching to help your body relax and then observe your thoughts. To each scary contribution your mind makes, add the observation 'It is what it is. I accept this.'

Fear of dying

Acceptance is particularly useful for dealing with the thought that trumps all other fears. It usually sounds something like this:

I AM GOING TO DIE!

I was fascinated to learn that the Buddhist tradition includes meditating on death. To most of us from a western background this seems like a morbid and depressing thing to do. Who would want to sit and contemplate their own death?

Then you realise that meditating on death sounds very different to being terrified of death. It sounds like this:

Everything that lives must die. I am going to die.

Can you recognise the difference? The first one screams at us and sends us into a tailspin. The second is just a statement of fact.

For some of us, death is already close. If you have received the news that there's no further treatment you can be offered, that your cancer has metastasized and that your options are palliative then fear of death is both real and pressing.

If you're not in this situation it might seem cruel or inappropriate for me to be suggesting that anyone in this situation should contemplating their impending death, but friends with end stage cancer have reassured me that this is both beneficial and life affirming. It helps them to release their fear and make the most of each precious day.

Some tell me they are at peace with the idea of their death, and that learning to make room for their fear has helped them to achieve this.

What a wonderful thing to not spend your last months, or weeks, or days feeling sick with worry, but enjoying the people and the things you love.

That's not to say you won't have moments of fear, or even terror. You're human. Fear is normal. But you can make room for that fear, observe it, honour it and then get back to making the most of you life.

Here's an exercise to help you understand what I mean by accepting your most terrifying fear:

Activity: But not today

- When the fear of death starts to appear, take a moment. Breathe into your fear and recognise the difference between you, right here and now, and your thoughts.

- Repeat your fear and add the phrase 'What will be will be' or 'It is what it is' or 'I accept this.'

- Notice any impact this has on your fear of dying.

- Now add the phrase 'but not today', so your thought now sounds something like this: 'I am going to die. I accept this. It is what it is. I am going to die but not today.'

- Reconnect to your surroundings and notice your fear. It's likely it will hang around (this particular fear is a sticky one!) but that you also feel a calm acceptance around it.

Notice how this acknowledges the validity of your fear of dying but also reminds you that you still have today to enjoy life and make the most of it.

Be careful with this one. Done properly it acknowledges your fears as legitimate and reasonable, but it can also feel like you're arguing with yourself. If that's the case then let this one go and try something else.

It seems an odd gift for cancer to give us, but this appreciation of our own mortality might just be the best thing to come out of our illness.

People who act as if they are immortal take terrible risks with their health. They waste time on things that are unimportant or unproductive because they believe they will always have more time.

One of the surprising thoughts that calms me is the knowledge that, as I age, I am increasingly at risk of dying from any one of the common causes of human death, including heart attack or stroke.

This has always been true. I accept this.

And yet, I do not spend any time at all being fearful about heart attacks or strokes. I don't ignore these risks. I do what I reasonably can to minimise them. The reason this thought is calming is it's proof I can live with a very real, genuinely frightening risk (of strokes and heart attacks) and still have a joyful life. That's what I was doing before my cancer diagnosis.

The difference now is that I accept my death as inevitable and I live my life accordingly. I take much better care of my health and I value my time. I am much more discerning about how I spend my days, and who I spend them with, than I was before.

Acceptance is also a useful technique for dealing with chronic pain.

Activity: Making room for pain

I don't know many people who have come out the other side of cancer treatment without pain. Depending upon our age and whatever else we have going on, many people are also dealing with chronic pain caused by injury, illness or something degenerative like arthritis.

I'm in my fifties and the bone scans I had during treatment revealed some arthritis in my lower back. I also have ongoing issue with pain across my chest (and sometimes my back) as a consequence of a bilateral mastectomy.

When I was sent home from hospital I was given heavy-duty painkillers and at three months post-recovery my doctor prescribed them again. He told me I would probably need to take them for the rest of my life. Given the risks and side effects of the medication I was concerned, but also not prepared to endure chronic pain.

My pain is now well managed without any medication. I do yoga at home every day and attend one class a week. I have massage with an oncology specialist. I also use this activity.

- Sit comfortably with your hands in your lap and your eyes closed.

- Take five calming breaths.

- Imagine a light or a scan that starts at the top of your head and moves through your body. It moves slowly, carefully searching for any kind of pain and providing a healing light as it travels.

- When you notice any pain in your body, stop the light or scan at that place. Explore the pain with your mind. See if you can find the edges of it. Think how you would describe this pain. Is it sharp or dull? Throbbing or constant? You might get the impression of cold or heat, or of a particular colour, but you might not.

- Breathe into the pain and imagine your body expanding around it. Make room for the pain. Turn up the healing intensity on your light or scan and imagine it flooding into the pain.

- You might feel some relief from the pain and you might not. Both are fine. Just sit with the pain for a while, make room for it and fill it with healing energy.

- Continue this way through your entire body, stopping at any point where you find pain.

- When you reach the soles of your feet, imagine the healing energy of that light or scan moving slowly and smoothly back through your body and out the top of your head.

I've noticed many times that only some of my pain is related to injury or inflammation. The rest is my body clenching against the pain or trying to compensate for it. This exercise allows me to relax my body and I often feel less pain once I've finished (but not always).

Accepting my pain and making room for it has a noticeable impact. I not only experience less physical pain but I can often reduce my pain just by paying attention to it and breathing into it.

This method won't always result in the ability to take less pain medication and I'm not advocating that anyone put up with chronic pain. The stress of it is not good for you.

What you may notice is that you need less pain medication, or that you just feel more comfortable on it. Both are good results.

You will have probably already noticed that, once again, this is the opposite of using distraction. You're actually focusing intentionally on your pain.

That's not to suggest keeping busy with something you enjoy won't help you to manage pain. It will. But distraction will probably be far more effective once you've relaxed your body and let your mind know that you're paying attention to those very important pain signals.

Naming the emotion

The final exercise for acceptance works with any kind of emotion. It's also so simple it can be difficult for people to appreciate its effectiveness without trying it.

The next time you're feeling an uncomfortable emotion, or some physical sensation in your body causes you to suspect you are not getting in touch with your emotions, try this.

- Sit quietly and close your eyes. Take a few calming breaths.

- Name your emotions.

That's it. Just give them a name. I'll give you an example of how this one works. Recently we took the difficult decision to end the life of a darling old cat who had been part of our lives for 19 years.

Smooge was a rescue kitten and had brain damage and a range of other health problems, but he was a hugely affectionate cat. In the weeks before his death he developed renal problems and he deteriorated quickly. We chose to end his life before his symptoms became acute and distressing. We will miss him.

I've owned cats my whole adult life. This is not the first time I have made this awful but necessary choice. In the past I have always consoled myself with the knowledge that any cat we have owned has been loved and very well cared for.

I have told myself it is much kinder to do what is best for a pet, rather than selfishly sustaining their lives because we know how much we will grieve. I have comforted myself with the knowledge that I have spared further suffering.

I certainly had all these thoughts on the day we took Smooge to the vet. Then I remembered to practice my skills for dealing with difficult emotions. Instead of rationalising his death, I just sat with my emotions for a while.

I felt sad. When I felt it, instead of having a polite argument with myself I simply acknowledged the emotion. 'Here is sadness.' I cried. I spoke to my husband about feeling sad.

We held Smooge and talked to him while the vet gave him an injection. He was already sedated and I don't know how much he was aware of, but it helped us to soothe him. We brought him home and buried him in the garden. I felt sad.

When I woke the next day, I still felt sad, but not at all distressed. In the past it has taken me a long time to recover from the death of a pet. This time around was different. I suppose it's just possible that after being through this so many times I have become more accepting of the simple reality that owning pets means saying goodbye to them, but I believe the key was accepting my emotions honestly, and without judgment.

You might find that when you first start naming your emotions it's a surprisingly difficult thing to do. Depending upon your background (and to some extent, your gender) you might struggle to describe how you're feeling. If all else fails, use BLAH!

Sometimes when I'm anxiously waiting for a doctor to see me, feeling better is as simple as saying *here is fear* or *here is anxiety* or *there is blah.*

Accepting that things are as they are allows me to make room for whatever emotions bubble up. I can also relish the happy times. *here is joy*, *there is delight.*

Acceptance frees me up from judging my emotions. Over time I've become better at naming them. I can distinguish between sadness, melancholy and grief. I can appreciate the many flavours and degrees of joy. My emotions are no longer a messy bucket of something mildly embarrassing to be hidden from view. They are the sound track to my life, helping me to fully experience each event for what it is.

Be present and mindful

Most of us have three distinct conscious states.

The first is a kind of automatic pilot. We move through our day, completing routine tasks without the need to give them our full attention. Our mind is free to think of other things provided we allocate just a portion of our attention.

Most people recognise this state. It's the one that allows you to have a conversation, listen to music or zone out while you drive a car. It's the one that lets you cook dinner, or mow the lawn, while you plan your weekend or daydream about your next holiday. It's also the state you're in when your fears and concerns are occupying most of your attention while you go about your day-to-day activities.

The second state is one where we escape reality. If you've ever been completely transported by a good book or an exciting movie then you'll recognise this one. You might also be carried away by music or some kind of physical activity. Your mind can take you on a journey, just by harnessing the power of your imagination.

This state can be a very useful way to give your mind a bit of a holiday from whatever has been concerning you. It's sometimes a useful way to break a worry cycle, where even though you think you've moved on from something your mind keeps returning to it like a dog with a bone. Facing your fears is a very effective management strategy but you don't need to practice it every hour of every day.

The third is that state where we are completely focused on the real world and what is right in front of us. You've probably experienced this when you're working on something that requires your full attention or when something moves you emotionally, like the feeling you get when you're kissing someone you love and your full attention is on the connection between you. This state is known as mindfulness.

All these conscious states are useful. Our ability to do one thing while thinking about another, to be transported away from the everyday, or to be completely present and focused, have different benefits at different times.

The problem is we tend to get into the habit of doing one thing while thinking about another. That's not a problem when we're doing something routine, but we can wind up missing out on the joy of life if it becomes our default setting.

Have you ever had that experience where you've drifted off while you were driving the car? Something happens and you're suddenly focused on driving again. Hopefully the 'something' isn't an accident, but it's often a near miss.

Have you ever faced the frustration of a friend or partner who's trying to tell you something while your mind is busy doing something else? We can get so used to doing one thing with our body and another with our mind it becomes a pattern. The risk is we miss out on the things that really matter to us.

Mindfulness can be a misleading term. Our minds usually feel full. They sometimes feel so full we wonder how we'll cope if we have to use them for anything else. They jump from one thought to the next or obsessively chew over the same thought in a process known as 'rumination' (the same thing a cow does when it re-chews its food). This is not mindfulness.

Buddhists have a lovely name for that state where our minds jump from one idea to the next and back again. They call it 'the monkey mind'. Mindfulness is a state where you focus on the present moment rather than the future or the past. When you are learning mindfulness you can notice the monkey jumping around but he doesn't hold your attention for long. You can let him go.

Mindfulness teaches you to give your attention to what is right in front of you, without judging it as 'good' or 'bad'. You are curious, open to whatever occurs.

I think learning acceptance first makes it much easier to practice mindfulness. Acceptance is its foundation. If you've already been spending some time learning acceptance then you're half way to mindfulness.

We don't need to be mindful all the time. There is still great enjoyment to be had in curling up with a book or a movie. There are also times when it can be useful to deliberately use our ability to take our mind elsewhere while we do something mundane. The point of learning mindfulness techniques is really to help us increase our awareness. Each of our conscious states has benefits and we can amplify these if we are making a deliberate choice about which one we'd like to use.

You may have already practiced some mindfulness techniques. They've become very popular. I've had them recommended to me by a number of different health professionals during my treatment. Maybe you did too.

There's no doubt some people find them very helpful, all on their own. I didn't. I now understand why. I was using mindfulness as a form of distraction. When fear came up I would try to calm my mind with a relaxation recording or a breathing exercise and, at least in the short-term, I would sometimes feel a bit better.

But most of the time I really didn't. Most of the time it was like having someone talk to me over loud music. I couldn't really give either my full attention. I'd listen to someone use their soothing voice to suggest I clear my mind and my mind would respond with 'well, if I could do that, I wouldn't need you!'.

No matter how many times I listened to these recordings, I felt like I was having an argument with myself.

Now this makes sense. I hadn't acknowledged and faced my fear so my mind resisted all attempts to calm it down. That's why being present and mindful is here, in this part of the book. These techniques are very powerful, but only if you've already faced your fear.

If you rolled your eyes with skepticism at the title of this chapter because of your previous poor experiences with meditation or mindfulness then please take a moment to consider this. Maybe your problem was context. Now you've developed some skills in making room for your emotions you might have a different experience with mindfulness.

So, if we've already learned how to face our fears, why bother with mindfulness? Do you remember what I wrote about the mind's ability to lay down tracks and to repeat patterns of behaviour? These are called neural pathways. Your mind makes it easy to find things it considers useful by establishing physical connections in your brain. Scientists used to think adult human brains were pretty much static but they now know we have 'neural plasticity'. This means we can form new neural pathways and replace old ones.

Essentially we can alter the way we think.

Your mind has probably become very good at scaring you. It's done that because the stakes are high. Cancer can be fatal and you know that only too well. Your mind has probably developed some excellent and highly creative strategies for frightening you and has then reinforced those neural pathways so it can keep doing that efficiently. (What a good mind it is to be making your survival such a priority.)

The trouble is cancer is not like a savage animal or an attacking human, and learning to be afraid of yourself and your own mind sets you into a downward spiral. Interestingly, it can also contribute to chronic pain. Being in a constantly heightened state of fear starts to cause physical changes in your brain. Those physical changes make you much more susceptible to physical pain.

Mindfulness can heal you. It can reduce the stress hormones that accumulate in your system and keep the release of them for times when you really need them. Better yet, some mindfulness techniques, like meditation, can actually help to restructure your brain so you are less likely to feel fear, anxiety and even physical pain.

This is about so much more than just being calm.

So even if you've tried and dismissed mindfulness or meditation in the past, please give it a try. Ideally, this should become a regular habit and finding 10 or 15 minutes each day will reward you with a huge return on your investment.

The present

I've called this section 'be present and mindful' because a part of every useful exercise in mindfulness is some component of becoming present, of not being lured by past memories or imaginings of future events but to be right here, right now, in the present moment.

You can't be mindful without being present. It's the state where all of you shows up. You're not compiling shopping lists or figuring out your budget. You're not digging up the past. It is possible to meditate in ways that carry you off into the realms of your imagination. They can be very enjoyable but they are different to the kind of meditations that help you to be present and mindful.

Becoming present is a good strategy for improving your relationships with others, your engagement with any activity you want to undertake and your ability to achieve your goals. I think the main reason to cultivate 'presence' is that it allows you to enjoy your life so much more.

I can sit opposite my daughter at lunch and really listen to what she has to share with me. I can give my husband my undivided attention and enjoy the glow it gives him when I do. Being present for the people I love benefits all of us.

When you've had cancer, becoming present also helps you to let go of the fear that lives in your past and that you imagine in your future. I know people who have been told there is nothing more medical science can do for them. Becoming present and mindful has given them a way to cherish each and every day they have left.

There are times when being present will mean dealing with the fear that's in front of you. It could be that your day includes bad news or a new symptom. Even then, being mindful and present can be a good thing.

By processing a real and present fear, acknowledging your emotional response to it and connecting to what matters in your life you'll be demonstrating to your mind that you have a real appreciation of the risks. This will reduce the need for your mind to keep reminding you. You will also help to avoid post-traumatic stress disorder because you have processed your emotions in real time, rather than parking them in the hope you will somehow process them later.

It's been difficult for me to get my head around the idea that my problems with post-traumatic stress stemmed from a desire to look brave and strong in circumstances where I was honestly horrified and appalled. Now I know that the people who don't develop this disorder feel the same way I did. The difference is they named those feelings, made room for them and did their job anyway. Mindfulness might just be the best defense against this kind of trauma.

Since learning how to face my fears I've realised for many of us, including me, it's not possible to be mindful until I've dealt with my emotional state in a healthy way. It's certainly impossible for me to meditate when I'm in the grip of fear. Please keep that in mind as you try these exercises. It could be that you need to revisit an early section of this book before you proceed.

What is meditation

Meditation is not the only way to learn mindfulness, but it's one of the best known.

Mention meditation and most people imagine someone sitting in a lotus position, chanting or counting their breathing or attempting to attain some kind of transcendental state – and meditation certainly can be all of these, but it is so much more. In its simplest form, meditation is training your mind to pay attention to just one thing. It does not need to have a religious context (but it can if you wish) and it does not require any special techniques or equipment.

Even if you've never learnt meditation, you've almost certainly had some experience of it. Have you ever been so engaged in an activity that time seemed to become distorted. It either felt like it had stopped, or you looked up from something you'd been enjoying only to realise it was many hours later than you thought. Both of these experiences are simple forms of meditation.

When my daughter was born I sat in bed holding her and gazing down at her in complete wonder and awe. This tiny, precious human had grown inside my body. I had been waiting a long time to meet her. She had my full and undivided attention for several hours as I simply gazed at her. My mind found this so enjoyable and so restful that I did not need sleep.

When I first learnt to paint with watercolours I found it challenging and sometimes frustrating to attempt a picture. There was a gap between what I wanted to do with the paint and what I was actually able to do. I practiced and over time the gap started to close. One day I looked up from a painting, deeply happy with the results, and realised I had missed lunch and dinner while I was painting.

This is a state known as 'flow', when you are so focused on something that it captures your complete attention. It's unlike any other feeling. It's deeply connected to what really matters to you. It's like a holiday for your mind. Practicing meditation can give you this kind of experience regularly.

Having a single point of focus is the beginner level of meditation. It's also possible to reach a state where you transcend your mind and body and experience deep and profound connection to all living things. There is no shortcut for achieving this and it can take years.

It's not my intention to teach you any techniques for higher-level meditation but I like to let people know there is more to it than having a single point of focus if they'd like to pursue further training.

For now, I'd like to focus on the benefits it can bring to those of us recovering from cancer and dealing with fear. Meditation can help you to feel calmer, to rewire your brain so it operates more effectively and to respond to all of your emotions in healthy ways. It can also help you to connect to the here and now, and to live each day fully.

Add to that, the proven ability of meditation to rewire your neural pathways and rebuild your prefrontal cortex and you're getting a lot of benefits from a very simple practice.

Surely that's worth 10 minutes a day.

Activity: Meditation on the breath

This meditation is one of the easiest to learn and practice. Remember, it's not a way to face your fears but something to do after you've faced them.

- If it's at all possible, find somewhere private to sit down. You want to be comfortable but not so comfortable that you'll fall asleep. Sitting in an office chair or a kitchen chair works well for most people. You can also sit on the floor if that suits you.

- **Close your eyes** and tilt your chin down slightly. Let your hands rest comfortably in your lap.

- **Take a slow, deep breath in**. Pay attention to the way the air feels coming in through your nose. Feel your belly and your chest expand.

- Once you've taken a deep breath in, hold it for a moment and then gently let the air escape from your body. Don't try to force your breath out. Just **exhale fully**. Keep exhaling until you feel like your lungs are empty.

- Now take **five more breaths**. With each one count slowly as you inhale and count slowly as you exhale. Notice how your breath feels as it enters and leaves your body. Observe it without judgment, the way you might observe a breeze moving through the trees. Notice the air feels slightly cooler on your inhale and slightly warmer on your exhale.

- Try to **make your exhale just a bit longer than your inhale**. You might like to use a phrase like 'I am breathing in', followed by 'and now I am going to breathe out all the way'. Say these phrases very slowly to yourself as you breathe. Keep noticing the air moving in and out of your body.

- While you're taking these five breaths, let whatever thoughts occur to you come and go in their own time.

- **Notice your thoughts but don't grab onto them**. Your thoughts might hang around or drift away. Both are fine. They are just thoughts. If you find your mind drifting, just gently move your attention back to your breathing.

- When you've taken your five breaths, open your eyes and look at where you are.

- **Notice** your hands and your body. Feel your clothing against your skin and your body against the chair or seat.

- **Notice** what's around you. The sights, the smells the sounds.

- **Notice** the temperature. The time of day. What is it about the place where you are that captures your attention?

Did this activity seem strangely familiar to you? Bonus points if you recognised it as a modified version of taking a moment and full marks if you've just figured out that you've already been meditating for weeks.

All of the activities I've given you so far involve elements of meditation. Of course, the previous activities had a specific purpose. They were designed to help you face your fears and come back into the present moment. Not all meditations will offer you this.

Two of my favorite meditations are variations of 'leaves on a stream' and 'clouds in the sky'. I close my eyes and use either analogy to relax my mind. If you enjoyed these activities when you were facing your fears you might like to try them as meditation exercises. You just use exactly the same visualisation but now you do it as a regular daily practice, regardless of how you're feeling.

Or you might like something new, like this next one.

Activity: The ball of light

- Sit somewhere comfortable with your hands in your lap and close your eyes.

- Imagine a bright, radiant ball of light. You might imagine it as being like the sun, or a bright jewel like a diamond, or an orb of light. Imagine it floating in front of your face and becoming as small as the tip of your nose.

- Imagine the light travelling up one nostril and filling your nose with light. Feel it radiate health.

- Imagine the light travelling to the middle of your brain and expanding to fill your skull. Feel it radiate health and calm.

- Imagine the light moving down to your throat and filling your throat with light. Feel it radiating health, calm and safety.

- Imagine the light moving down to your chest and filling your chest cavity with light. Feel it radiating health, calm, safety and love.

- Imagine the light moving down to the space behind your navel and filling your lower body with light. Feel it radiating health, calm, safety, love and energy.

- Sit with this feeling for a while and then allow the light to grow inside you and to flood your entire body with health, calm, safety, love and energy.

- Open your eyes and come back into the room (or space). Notice your surroundings as if you are seeing them for the first time.

This one is easy to learn and practice. Read through it a few times and then try it. You don't need to get too caught up with the script. You're just imagining a light moving through various parts of your body and you're adding a word at each stop. You can substitute other words if you don't like these ones. You can also adapt the words to particular situations.

I have a friend who uses it before she performs on stage as a violinist to calm her nerves and she uses words like agility, focus, joyfulness, presence and excellence.

I've had people tell me they can't meditate because they have chronic pain and this keeps pulling them out of any attempt. Meditation can work with what you've got.

You might like to return to the previous activity 'making room for pain' and try it as a meditation. Or you could try something new, like this one:

Activity: Clenching and unclenching

If you've ever attended yoga classes you will probably be familiar with this meditation. It uses the clenching of muscles to make you conscious of how your body is feeling.

It's also good for pain management but you don't need to be in pain to find it useful. This one appeals particularly to anyone who finds visualisation difficult or a bit too 'out there'. You don't need to imagine anything with this one.

- Find somewhere comfortable and lay on your back (you can also do this one seated, but it works better if you're stretched out flat).

- Take your attention to your feet. Clench the muscles in your feet as tightly as you can. Curl your toes in and see how tight you can make your muscles. Breathe in while you do this.

- Exhale and relax your feet. Feel all the tension leave your feet at the same time your breath leaves your body.

- Take another breath in and clench your calf muscles. As you exhale, release the tension and let those muscles relax.

- Now repeat the process with your thigh muscles. Clench them as tightly as you can on the inhale and relax them as you exhale.

- Work your way up your body, clenching different muscle groups. If you prefer you can work either side of you body separately, or you can start at your head and move downwards. All that matters is that every muscle is clenched and released.

- As you release each muscle group you might like to think of a word or a phrase like 'letting go' or 'release' (but you don't have to).

- Once you have worked your way around your entire body, clench all the muscles on the right hand side and then release them.

- Now clench all the muscles on the left hand side and then release them.

- Clench your whole body and take a deep breath while you do. Hold the clench for as long as you can comfortably hold your breath. Exhale and release the tension in your body. See how long you can make your exhale.

- Finally, take five calming breaths and notice the difference in the way your body feels.

This meditation can be very useful if you're having trouble falling asleep at night. It's also a good way to locate and release pain. You may find you have less pain at the end of this meditation and you may find your pain level is about the same, but because the rest of your body is relaxed the pain is easier to manage.

Any meditation can help with pain because you'll be helping to rebuild the part of your brain known as the prefrontal cortex. This area is smaller in people who experience chronic pain. Meditation, practiced over time, strengthens the prefrontal cortex and helps it to return to a healthy size. So if you don't particularly like a pain-specific meditation, any other meditation can still help.

If you have issues with pain why not try a short meditation each day for a couple of weeks and see how you feel. You might find you can give up pain medication after a while, and you might find you can reduce it. It could be you will need the same amount of pain relief but meditation will still help you to live well and make room for the pain.

Like all of these techniques, meditation requires a bit of time and a bit of practice. When I was learning to meditate, I found it useful to link it to my existing routine. I never forget to shower or clean my teeth so using these events to remind myself to practice facing my fear along with being present and mindful made sense. You might like to do the same.

It's also worth knowing it's possible to become mindful and present without closing your eyes and visualising. Some people find this type of activity preferable to meditation. Here's an example of one of these activities. Why not try it and see what you think?

Activity: Eating mindfully

- Choose a food you enjoy. You don't need a lot of it. Just a taste. It might be a slice of apple or a strawberry. You might prefer a cube of your favourite cheese or a spoonful of ice cream.

- Put that food in your mouth and give it your undivided attention. What does it taste like? What sort of texture does it have? Does it change as you hold it in your mouth?

- Notice what you are doing with your mouth. Are you chewing? Where is the food in your mouth? What part is your tongue playing in the process? Are you swallowing all the food at once or are you taking your time?

- Notice the after-taste once you've swallowed the food. How does your mouth feel? Is it warmer or colder than it was before? Or does it feel the same? Is there anything stuck in your teeth or has every part of the food been swallowed.

How did you go? You might have noticed when you gave your full attention to eating something your mind calmed down and you didn't have any intrusive thoughts. You may have noticed you still had unrelated thoughts drifting through your mind but your focus on eating allowed them to just appear and then float off in their own time.

Our minds like to be busy. Interestingly, recent research has found that worry will actually set off the reward centres in our brains. Yes, our brains are designed to physically reward us for worrying! It seems that even worry is better than doing nothing, but giving our minds something else to focus on is definitely preferable to worry.

This might be why mindfulness exercises can work really well, all on their own, for some people. If you're a worry addict then mindfulness gives your mind a better option.

Eating mindfully has also been shown to help people that overeat. Focusing on each mouthful of food helps them to slow down and to appreciate their meal. It gives the receptors in their body the time to register that they're feeling full. It also helps to calm the mind and to reduce the tendency some people have to overeat when they are worried.

Mindful eating is a very specific, focused activity that requires you to stop what you're doing and focus on just one thing, but there's an even easier form of mindfulness that can help you to be more present.

Activity: Becoming present

- Wherever you are and whatever you're doing, stop and take a moment. Practice holding yourself gently and breathing. Observe your mind generating thoughts but use the techniques you've been practicing to just acknowledge that those thoughts exist and to let them float away in their own time.

- Open your eyes if you closed them and start noticing your body and the things around you. Examine everything around you in close detail using as many of your senses as possible. What can you see, hear, touch, taste and smell? Imagine you're a police officer conducting an investigation and you're looking for clues. Observe everything in detail.

- Return to your day but with that same focus on the world around you and your place in it. Notice how your body feels and where it comes into contact with the floor or your chair. Notice all of the physical things around you.

- Take some time to really listen to the sounds you usually ignore. What is their source? Pay attention to the quality of the light, any breeze or air movement, the look and texture of the details around you.

- Notice the difference between you in your environment and the thoughts that are happening in your mind. When your mind tries to distract you, acknowledge the thought without trying to push it away. (You might like to say something like 'here is another thought' or you might just label it 'thought') and then refocus on the present.

This type of exercise is sometimes called a moving meditation. It's interesting when you're learning this activity to observe how easily your attention will drift away. This is normal. Most people find they can only remain present for a few minutes at most before they start being pulled into the past or the future by their mind.

And yes, this one is also a rework of something from the section on facing your fears (see what I did there?).

Part of the strength of this exercise is the way it makes us much more aware of our usual state of mind. We usually understand that being present and giving what's happening in our life right now our full attention makes sense. How do we get the most out of life if we're not in it? And yet when we try to remain present it can be shocking to discover how difficult it is.

Be gentle with yourself. Being present and mindful are worthy goals and worth your time and effort but if you start to beat yourself up you're not likely to achieve either. Self-bullying is usually a voice from the past. It encourages us to judge ourselves by past failures or to give up before we've even tried.

When my mind starts to do this I find this idea really useful. Every cell in my body is renewing itself. Some, like the cells in my blood, are doing this relatively quickly while others, like bone cells, are doing it more slowly, but every single cell is renewing itself.

In addition to my cells renewing, every day brings me new opportunities, new experiences and new things to learn. This means I am not the person I was yesterday. I am certainly not the person I was five years ago and I can see obvious changes between who I am today and who I was in the past the further back I go.

By observing this pattern I can conclude that the person I am today is not the person I will be tomorrow. I will be slightly different. In five years' time I am likely to be significantly different, both in terms of my cellular make-up and my mind.

This means the stories my mind is telling me about the past relate to a different version of me. I am not that person. The stories my mind tells me about the future me are stories about someone I may or may not become, but I am not yet that person.

There is one other activity I'd like you to try for becoming mindful and present. It will also help you to rewire your brain, calm your noisy fears and improve your life on a daily basis. Like meditation, you have probably already heard of this one.

Activity: Being genuinely grateful

Gratitude is sometimes prescribed for dealing with fear and some people find it does help, but I think it's most effective when you don't use it as a distraction. Even though it's a very pleasant distraction it doesn't give your mind any sense of being heard and understood.

So please use it in addition to facing your fears rather than as an alternative.

- Choose one day each week to record things you are genuinely grateful for.

- On that day, make a record of seven things and the reason you are grateful for each one. The way you record them doesn't matter.

- Try not to repeat anything. Ideally you should come up with seven new things each week.

- Find things you are **genuinely** grateful for. Take some time to really think about what it is in your life that inspires gratitude.

Suggestions for recording include keeping a journal, posting seven photographs to social media, putting them on post-it notes where you can see them or pairing up with someone else and exchanging your thoughts each week.

Some people form gratitude groups where everyone shares their reasons for feeling grateful but you can just as easily do this on your own.

Some people prefer to do this daily, but the research has shown that doing it just once a week and noticing seven things is much more effective. I think that's because it puts you back into a grateful state of mind several times, all through the week. It can be relatively easy to put just one thing in a journal each night, but finding seven things once a week needs a bit more effort and thought.

I first started doing this because my daughter challenged me to post seven photos each week. She did the same. The challenge was supposed to go for a year but she became too busy with her university studies. I switched to posting seven statements about things I was grateful for each week and most weeks I still do, even more than five years after I first started doing it.

What I've noticed is that making a record of the things I am grateful for each week makes me more mindful and present for the whole of the week. I'm not just passively noticing the world around me. I'm actively hunting for things to appreciate.

The consequence of keeping this record for several years has been the creation of some pretty robust neural networks for gratitude. I can't prove this process has rewired my brain, but I feel certain it has.

I now feel a much deeper appreciation for all the people in my life and for everything I own. My gratitude extends to the people who have invented or created the things I use, for the earth and all life on it, for the weather and the seasons and for being fortunate enough to live in a country with clean running water. I don't just feel this on Sunday, when I make my list, but all through the week.

I was born into a family of critical thinkers. We would spend our evenings debating and dissecting the world and the people in it. I became acutely judgmental as a consequence. Not a bad training ground for a future police officer but not particularly useful in my personal relationships.

Now I value my husband's compassion and intellect and wonder at my daughter's fine moral compass and generous heart. It's not that they don't have any flaws, but that my perspective is to approach both of them with gratitude rather than judgment. I have also developed the ability to be grateful for my own good qualities and less critical of myself. I wonder if people who aren't acutely judgmental realize that those of us made this way are harshest on ourselves.

Establishing a practice for expressing gratitude can make a big difference in your life, eventually. This isn't like lifting weights or taking up running. The changes are slow and subtle.

It's possible at this point that some part of you is wondering where you are going to find the time for all these new activities. Please know that everything in this book can be achieved in less than 10 minutes a day. You might want to take a little bit longer, or even much longer, just because you're finding the activities enjoyable. But 10 minutes will work too.When you consider all the benefits available to you, 10 minutes isn't too difficult to find.

I have a final caution for the gratitude exercise. If it feels like it's becoming competitive, you're doing it wrong. It's not an opportunity to boast about all the nice stuff you own or to exhibit your wealth. You're not trying to prove you're the fittest, most attractive, most talented or most accomplished person on the planet. You're not even trying to prove you're the kindest or the most grateful.

That's why this section is about being **genuinely** grateful.

Other ways to be mindful and present

I'm hoping you have already understood that distraction alone won't necessarily be effective against your fears. You're not paying attention to the warning signals your clever mind is sending you and so it's going to keep revisiting old territory.

Having said that, we now also know that a mind with nothing to do might resort to worry to stimulate the brain's reward centres. This is why some forms of distraction work some of the time. We're keeping our mind momentarily occupied. It's a bit like handing a toy to a bored child in a shopping trolley.

When you use the techniques in this book on a regular basis to take a moment and to face your fears, you'll calm your distressed mind. It's important once you've done that to give it something to keep it occupied so it doesn't use the default setting of worry out of habit.

Being mindful and present achieves this, and also helps you to get the most out of each day. Instead of just sending your body in while your mind is occupied, you learn to be fully present and to really connect to what matters. You also know that, over time, being present and mindful will physically change your brain. The neural networks that made worrying your default setting will gradually be replaced by a tendency to be present and mindful. Hooray!

Now that you have a better understanding of what it means to be mindful and present, here's a quick quiz. Which of the following activities do you think would involve being mindful and present?

Drawing or painting a picture

Writing in a journal

Going on a holiday

Taking a short course

Playing with a dog

Doing an exercise class

Laughing at something funny

How did you go?

The correct answer might be all of them, but it might be none of them. All of these activities can be done mindfully while being present, but it's not a requirement.

It's possible to do just about anything and still have fear screaming away in your head. This is not being mindful and present. Most of us have had this experience. It is distressing. Fear keeps us from connecting to what matters. We become a kind of fear zombie, going through the motions of our life but not really living.

Becoming mindful and present puts us back into our bodies and back into the real world. It's possible we can become so connected that our fear vanishes for a while. What a relief! It's also possible doing something mindfully just turns down the volume of our fear, so it's like a distant background noise that doesn't need our immediate attention. As long as we make sure to give it some attention, some of the time, this is also a good outcome.

Let's go through each of the examples in the quiz so you can see what I mean about all of them being opportunities for becoming mindful and present.

Drawing a picture might be a half-hearted attempt to escape fear or it might be a genuine attempt to express it. You will remember one of the previous activities gave you the opportunity to create a piece of art that represented your fear. This could be a useful mindfulness exercise.

You can also get creative just for the joy of it. If you enjoyed drawing or colouring-in, even if that was a long time ago, then drawing might be a great activity for your mindfulness and presence.

Try drawing something that's right in front of you to ramp up the effect. Remember, mindfulness requires you to let go of your judgment. Be curious and interested in the results of your efforts.

You can do the same thing with journaling by describing what is around you and above you and in front of you. Journaling about past and future events has its own benefits but you're not being present while you're doing that, particularly if you're writing about your cancer. If, however, you're completely engaged in creative writing, thinking about how best to express something, then this could well be an exercise in mindfulness.

Holidays can be a huge relief to your mind, provided your time is filled with new and interesting things to keep you engaged in the present moment. Many of us have our strongest experiences of being mindful and present while we're gazing at a natural or human-made wonder.

However, sitting around on holidays with nothing to do is likely to give your mind far too much spare time and there's a possibility you will fall back into chewing over the past. Remember: a mind with nothing to do may well resort to worry. That's not to say you can't relax in a deck chair, but do it in a way that connects you to your surroundings.

If you're planning a holiday consider how to amplify the opportunities for mindfulness and presence. You might like to include some kind of class or challenging activity. You might prefer to connect with the natural world. Figuring out what is most likely to help you achieve mindfulness will guarantee a much better break for both your mind and your body.

Taking a short course in something you've always wanted to learn, or to refresh knowledge you once had, will not only help you to be mindful and present but will have the added benefit of laying down new neural pathways. People recovering from brain injury and stroke are now given opportunities to learn a musical instrument or a new language for this reason.

I found several short courses online when I was recovering from the cognitive damage done by chemotherapy. I also attended some courses with other people and this really helped to get my brain firing again. I noticed when I'm learning something new I tend to give it my undivided attention. It's a great mindfulness shortcut for me.

Playing with a dog, or any other pet, can bring some people instantly back into the room and out of their minds. Animals have a wonderful capacity to capture our full attention. As I write this, the newest addition to our family, Harry, is purring away in my lap. Like all kittens, he is completely captivating.

As an extra benefit, cuddling your pet will release the feel-good hormone, oxytocin, into your system. So will nursing a baby (but please ask the parents first!). All human beings crave physical contact and our endocrine system rewards us when we get it.

If, on the other hand, you're worrying about who will care for your pet if something happens to you, or how much pet food is going to cost you this week, you are not being mindful and present.

So how about an exercise class?

Some forms of exercise are designed to build our ability to be mindful and present. The whole concept of mindfulness probably originates with yoga (it was apparently a yogi that taught Buddha). Don't be put off by the pretzel girls in lycra. When I started yoga I was 16 kilos overweight and I couldn't balance on one leg. If you can't get to a class there are now plenty of online yoga resources (and they're free).

Tai Chi, Qigong and some forms of martial arts also have a strong mindfulness component. It's possible to do any kind of exercise mindfully, but you can probably appreciate the difference between giving what you are doing your full attention and using it to keep your body busy while your mind ruminates.

And if you're still short of ideas for being mindful and present you might just need a good laugh.

Humour is a very special kind of mindfulness. We usually find something funny because of an unexpected connection or a surprise. Laughter fires off unrelated neural pathways and makes a tentative connection between them. It causes a cascade of beneficial reactions in our bodies that improve our mood and boost our immune system. It's good for our brains. It's also difficult to think of anything else when we are laughing. This might be why it has a reputation for being the best medicine.

You are mindful and present when you are finding something genuinely funny. That's different to trying to make a joke out of your legitimate fears.

I have a caution here regarding books, television and movies. We can read or watch mindfully but the very nature of these activities is that they take us out of the present. There's nothing wrong with books, movies or television but be aware they are not useful when you want to become present – except, of course, books like this one about being mindful and present.

When we read or watch events involving other people our brains actually fire as if the same events are happening to us. This can be a wonderful thing for building empathy and developing tolerance. It's also why you should avoid things that are threatening or frightening for a while.

If you feel like escaping from your present circumstances then fiction can provide you with a kind of mental holiday, taking your mind on wonderful imaginary journeys. Just be a bit careful with the destinations you choose.

I watched a lot of children's movies during treatment. They were funny, reliably enthralling and they always had a happy ending. I avoided thrillers, heavy drama and horror movies. I had enough of those in my day-to-day life.

It's also a good idea to be aware of those activities that are just like riding a bike. Riding a bike is a reasonably challenging activity. The hormones released if we do it are good for us, but this is an example of an activity that can become automatic. We get familiar with the bike and the surroundings and, if we're not careful, our minds float off to the land of fear.

Any activity we're familiar with can become just like this. It can require more and more effort to anchor ourselves in the present and to avoid automatic pilot. If you find this happening when you're seeking mindfulness then try a new activity. Alternatively, tune into your surroundings. Take your bike somewhere new and enjoy the change. Connect to the outside world.

Remember, you don't need to be competitive with anyone. Choose a mindfulness activity for the joy of it. Competition is something else that pulls you out of the present because you're only thinking about the outcome and not enjoying the process. Competing with yourself can also drag you out of the present because you'll be using an old version of yourself as your reference point.

I've only given you a handful of examples but I hope they've helped to clarify what I mean by being mindful and present. You don't need to meditate if it doesn't appeal to you. You can just shift your attention to becoming more mindful and present in your everyday activities.

You may have noticed when you're feeling really frightened you can experience a heightening of your senses, thanks to the adrenaline and cortisol in your system. Your vision, smell and hearing are all enhanced. What a great opportunity to practice some mindfulness techniques and really take in the world around you.

You can also use gratitude to anchor you in the present moment. I can stand at the kitchen sink, doing the washing up and give my full attention to the dishes, the water and the foam from the detergent. I can feel grateful for running water, the meal I've just eaten and the people I've shared it with.

You probably don't really want to do nothing

There's a common misconception human beings enjoy doing nothing. I suspect this is a consequence of the marketing for various holidays that want to promote the benefits of spending a week in a deck chair. There are certainly times when all of us could benefit from a bit more relaxation but what research into human motivation tells us is that we are actually happiest when we have a challenge.

I read about this research while I was on a short cruise, wondering why I was feeling so bored. Turns out I'm not alone. This might be why they organise all those activities to keep people distracted on a cruise ship. I decided I would have rather done a short course somewhere. It seems finding something challenging to do is deeply satisfying no matter who you are.

There's a proviso to this. The challenge has to be enough to stretch us but not so difficult we feel overwhelmed or frustrated by it. We're also much more likely to enjoy a challenge if it's safe to make mistakes and we're not being forced or intimidated into participating.

Medical professionals understand this (at least the good ones do!). We respond better to the challenges of cancer treatment when we are given access to information, choices about treatment (where there are legitimate choices available) and the opportunity to give informed consent.

Many of us also figure out what the people who design popular computer games have realised. Human beings will be more motivated by things that are divided into manageable chunks. Did you get through chemotherapy by just focusing on the next infusion? Did you have times during treatment when your short-term goal was to just get through the week, or the day?

If so, you've figured out something that most people have in common.

One of the best ways to break up a challenging event in your life is to break it into pieces of time. (There's a good reason recovering addicts are told to just focus on one day at a time). When you put the effort into being mindful and present you're also achieving this. Your focus is on what you can do today.

That's not to say that you don't have long-term goals (more on that in the next section) but that you give your focus to what you can do right now.

When you're developing your skills at mindfulness and being present, start by just seeing if you can achieve one minute of focus on your present surroundings. Set goals each day to spend just a bit more time being mindful and present.

Learning these skills will reward you with a greater connection to what matters in your life. You won't miss the joy of what's around you because you're watching horror movies in your head or attending to the mundane.

Connection with other people is a primary need for all human beings. Fear can make us so hyper-vigilant we distance ourselves from others. Becoming mindful and present can help us start to reconnect again.

As you can see, while the benefits of meditation are undeniable, they are not the only way to achieve a calmer and more present mind. You can incorporate your new knowledge into your everyday activities. Sometimes it's as simple as just looking up from what you're doing and noticing the detail around you.

As a short exercise in mindfulness, why don't you try that now? Put down this book and just take in your surroundings for a few minutes. See how long it takes for other thoughts to start popping up, and when they do, resist the temptation to judge yourself or your thoughts. Just let them float on by.

I'm hoping that by this stage of the book you have developed some great skills for facing your fears and you have started exploring how you might be more mindful and present. There are only two more sections to go.

I've told you that mindfulness and presence will help you to focus on what really matters in your life but how do you figure out what that is? The next section is all about finding your focus and discovering the answers to that question.

Finding your focus

What was the best thing for you about getting cancer? To anyone who has never had it this seems like a strange question, but everyone I've met who has had cancer can answer this quickly and with a great deal of conviction.

Answers are personal, but are usually some variation of 'I figured out what really matters'. Here are some of the other answers I've heard:

I don't care what other people think about me any more. I have a much deeper appreciation of my family and friends.

I realised there are some things I really want to do with my life and I need to start doing them now. I've stopped procrastinating and started making better use of my time.

I've stopped treating my body as if I'm immortal. I've changed the way I eat and I now actually have an exercise routine.

I have let go of all my past hurts and I've forgiven the people who caused them. I realised that they were taking up time and energy that they didn't deserve and giving them so much attention was living in the past.

I've become an advocate for other people with cancer and I donate time to a charity every week. It's my way of giving back to all the people that supported me during treatment and I find it deeply satisfying.

I just don't sweat the small stuff. So may of the things I used to get wound up about just don't bother me anymore.

I realised that no amount of stuff will ever make me happy so now I have less stuff and I spend more time doing things I care about. I did a big clean out and gave a lot of stuff away. I don't spend money the way I used to. I save it for things that matter.

I know it's a cliché but love really is the only thing that matters.

I really think this is the silver lining of having survived cancer. Most of us experience a great deal of clarity about what matters most to us. I suspect we find identifying what really matters to us much easier than most people. Something about staring down death gives us that sort of clarity.

Good timing, because the next part of reclaiming your life from the fear monsters is to be very clear about your priorities, and how you want to live your best life. (Hooray!)

You've hopefully mastered some great techniques for facing your fear, acceptance and being mindful and present. Now you're ready to spend some time thinking about your future and how you want that to be. How will you decide what it is that matters most to you and what will you do about that once you know?

The pursuit of happiness

Books and programs on happiness and positivity have made their authors loads of money in recent years, and why not. Who wouldn't want to be happier? The problem is that happiness is not a perpetual state. Nobody is happy all the time.

We know even famous and wealthy people suffer from illness, divorce and death to at least the same extent as the rest of us. There's now even a spate of books on how to recover from the pressure some people feel to be happy all the time.

Happiness is not a permanent state. We all know this. It might be that you sometimes have one glorious day where you are happy for every waking hour but this would be, for most of us, a rare event. Like every other emotion, happiness comes in waves. So having happiness as your primary goal is guaranteed to leave you feeling disappointed.

The alternative is to focus instead on leading a **fulfilling life**, a life full of meaning and purpose and things that really matter to you. There's research showing that when you focus on leading a fulfilling life (rather than a simply happy one) you are much more likely to express satisfaction and contentment, and to have a sense of achievement, even if your circumstances are not always good.

The key to having a fulfilling life is to figure out what your values are, which ones matter most to you and then to take action that's consistent with those values.

When I first encountered this idea, it was immediately appealing to me. I knew, in spite of my best efforts, there had been many times throughout my life when I was dealing with something difficult or challenging. It was certainly impossible to be relentlessly happy during cancer treatment. My life included good days, bad days and some that were a bit of both. The same was true of everyone I had ever met.

I remember hearing the Dalai Lama respond to a question about an annoying neighbour. The person asking the question described some awful behaviour and asked for advice on how to avoid being angry. His Holiness replied, 'You can't. That would make me angry too.' Everyone in the auditorium laughed but it was an excellent point to make.

Even the Dalai Lama isn't happy all the time but his life is probably deeply fulfilling. That's because his values are very clear and he spends his entire life living them.

You don't need to be the reincarnation of a god to achieve this kind of peace. It's surprisingly easy.

What are values?

Your values define who you want to be as a person and what you want to stand for. When someone asks you 'what really matters to you?' your answers will directly reflect your values. Being clear about your values makes it much easier to live a fulfilling life because you can measure your progress against something that is genuinely meaningful to you.

A values-based life is the opposite of trying to impress other people or to meet their expectations. It's about finding that jewel of meaning that rests at the very heart of you, and being true to that.

Many of us share common values but we usually also have some that are less common. Most people value connection with others, for example, but only some crave the kind of excitement involved in extreme sports.

Here are some examples of what I mean by 'values':

Imagine you're a person who feels strongly about helping people. You take a job with a phone company that encourages you to use some fairly dubious tactics to sell phone plans and equipment to customers. Your performance is measured against the money you make and not against the satisfaction of the customers. You know you are selling people things they don't need. How do you feel?

It's likely you're very unhappy in this job. You're regularly acting in a way that's inconsistent with your values. Here's another scenario to illustrate what I mean:

You have applied for two different jobs. One of them pays a lot of money but requires you to do work that is mundane and boring. The other job doesn't pay as well but it's the type of work that you genuinely enjoy. Which job do you take? What influences your decision?

This is not an easy choice because the more enjoyable job might not give you enough of an income to meet your basic needs. It might not allow you to provide for other people you care about. You might take the higher paying job because you value financial security.

If you can meet your living expenses on the lower wage, and you value genuinely enjoyable work you would take the lower paying job. You might also consider altering some other aspect of your life so you can live on less money just so you could accept a more enjoyable job. It all depends upon your values.

Here's a scenario that isn't related to work. See what you think of this one:

You are single and interested in a couple of different people as prospective partners. One of them shares most of your hobbies and interests but has very different values to you – you value family and connection and they like to be independent; you value being frugal and saving money and they spend it as fast as they earn it. The other person has a lot of different hobbies and interests but shares your values. They also value family and connection and they are working towards financial security. Which person do you think will be the better partner?

This one is something that a lot of people don't consider at the start of a relationship, but I when you give it some thought the answer is obvious. Having common values is much more important than having similar interests. Sure, there needs to be some common ground when it comes to how you spend time together, but a major conflict in values is going to be a continuing source of distress to both of you.

Notice in this example that the values could have been reversed. It could be that you're a spontaneous person who likes to live in the present and saves only long enough to have the funds for your next adventure. You're probably also going to be better off with someone who shares those values, and you're certainly going to regularly come into conflict with someone who doesn't.

This is important. Values are personal. Just like emotions, they aren't good or bad. Having different values means we prioritise things differently.

Society also agrees on some common moral values, like not killing people or not stealing. These are different to your personal values (although for many of us there will be an alignment). Most of us want more out of life than to just avoid breaking the law or offending people.

Being clear about our values and using them to guide the decisions we make is at the heart of living a rich and fulfilling life. Here are some common examples of people living according to their values:

- A couple decides that time spent with their children is more important than wealth. They find work that pays less money so they can spend more time together as a family.

- Although an elderly couple appreciates the traditional view that property should be passed on to their children when they die, their strong values around philanthropy lead them to decide to leave a large proportion of their estate to their favorite charity.

- A person decides to spend their savings going travelling whenever they can afford it rather than investing in a home because they value the experiences that travel provides over home ownership.

- A person decides not to spend their savings on travel but to invest in a home because they value the security that property ownership provides.

- A person strikes a balance between spending money on travel and saving for a home because they value both.

As you can see, values are individual and vary from person to person. There's no one 'right' set of personal values and they can change over time or because of a change in our circumstances.

When we are younger we might value adventure and new experiences more highly that health and safety and we might take risks. As we get older we might still enjoy adventure, but place a higher value on family and safety.

Values are different to rules or strategies. A couple might decide that one of their strategies for building family connection is going on holidays together every year. The thing they value is 'family connection' and the thing they do about it is to go on holidays.

They might also have some rules about how family members will treat each other, like not taking someone else's property without asking or everyone helping with chores. The thing they value is still 'family connection' and the rules are an expression of that value.

Most families have lots of different rules and strategies designed to help everyone get along. All of these stem from their desire to have a good family life but the rules and strategies will vary enormously from family to family. Most of us have very strong opinions about the kind of family we want and we also accept that not everyone agrees with us.

Values apply to every aspect of our lives (not just families) but I like to use families as an example because most of us can relate to these. We all know that most families want very similar things when it comes to everyone getting along, but that they find many different rules and strategies for achieving them.

When we describe our values we usually use words like 'want' or 'desire' or 'aspire'. Rules tend to be described using words like 'must' or 'shouldn't'. A value is more of a guiding principle, a bit like the sky in the exercise you've learned. Strategies and rules become the clouds.

Understanding the difference between your values and what you do about them is important. It can be a major source of conflict. For example, one person in a family example might think that their best strategy is to work really long hours to earn lots of money to buy things, while the other might think that working shorter hours for less money is the way to go. Both of these people are motivated by their value around having a good family life but they have different ways of acting on it.

Here's a cancer-specific example to demonstrate my point:

Two survivors both share the same value. They both want to be as healthy as they can be following treatment. One of them decides to never drink alcohol again because they have read the research about alcohol and cancer. The other chooses to drink because they decide that sharing alcohol with friends is part of what makes their life enjoyable and that this connection contributes to their good health.

In this scenario you may have an opinion about who is right and who is wrong. In fact both choices are socially acceptable. Each person has made a decision based upon the same value (being healthy) but they appear to have made opposite choices. The point is that both people have found ways to live according to their values. Neither is 'right' or 'wrong'; they are just different.

This is the primary difference between personal values and social values. Most of us agree that it is wrong to kill people, or hurt them, or steal from them. These are moral values where there is strong agreement throughout our society regarding what is right and what is wrong. Social values do change over time but this change happens slowly. It took a long time for the laws to change regarding women voting or slavery being illegal. Both changes now reflect common social values.

Personal values are not as black and white and will change much more often. Here's an example.

Most people find their values around road safety suddenly undergo a big shift following the birth of their first baby. They are suddenly strongly supportive of police enforcing the road rules and they drive much more carefully now there's a baby in the car. Their values have changed.

Values are different to hopes and wishes. You might hope you win the lottery or that your partner becomes more loving. These are hopes about things beyond your control. Values are personal. They are about the kind of person you want to be. You can take action that is consistent with your values. True, you can buy a lottery ticket or let your partner know you'd like more affection, but the outcome of your actions is not up to you.

Your hopes and wishes can be helpful when you're defining your values. For example, your hope that your partner becomes more loving might be associated with your values around family and connection, or intimacy and support. Your desire to win the lottery might be associated with your values around financial security or independence.

Here is a handful of randomly selected values so you can see the kind of language used to describe them:

- Connection
- Excitement
- Safety
- Intimacy

All these values have been expressed as a single word. They can also be expressed as a sentence.

- I value connection with all living things
- I value connection with my close friends and family
- I value connection with a higher power

You can see that all these statements are different ways to express the value 'connection'.

There are pros and cons to using either words or sentences and you should feel free to play with both when you're putting together your own personal list of values. Sometimes I find a single word says it all for me, and other times I want to be clearer about what I mean.

I'm going to give you a couple of activities to help you to create a short list of your top values. These are just your most significant values for right now. Something might happen tomorrow to cause you to change them. There are no right answers. There are only answers that are right for you.

This is just a list of what matters most to you at this particular point in time. Nobody is going to hold you accountable to this list and it's not a tool for anyone's inner-bully to use as a weapon. So relax and have a bit of fun with this. If at the end of this chapter you don't like the five values you've selected, just throw them away and start again.

It's worth revisiting your values from time to time and seeing if they've changed. This can be particularly useful when you feel like your life is drifting off course or lacking meaning. It's a sure sign you're not living a life consistent with your values.

It's also a great activity after a major life event, like cancer treatment, because you've probably come out the other side of it with a much clearer idea about what really matters to you. Your values are about what you want to stand for in any given situation, and ultimately they're about what you want the whole of your life to represent.

Some people are very clear about their values but most of us need some help to identify them, and to decide which ones are the most important right now. Here are a couple of activities to help you get in touch with yours.

Activity: Admirable people

Thinking about the people we admire often gives us an insight into what really matters to us.

- Think of five people you admire and write down their names. They might be friends or family members. They might be famous or historical figures. The only requirement is that you find them admirable.

- Now write a short passage or a list of words about each person describing what you admire about them.

- Have a look at your descriptions of each person. Have you identified any of your own values?

The first time I did this exercise I included a wonderful woman I know called Glenys. She's in her 80s but inspires me with her passion for the environment and for social change. She is a deeply compassionate person who remains hopeful about the future. She helped me to get in touch with my values around caring for others and making a difference.

I also included my daughter, who is one of the kindest people I have ever met. She helps me to remember that nobody cares too much about whether my opinions are right or wrong if I am unkind in the way I express them.

I'm also inspired by people I've never met, like Douglas Adams and Sheri S Tepper (both authors) and David Attenborough.

It doesn't matter if the people you choose to admire are friends, family or famous. Just that you find something inspiring about them.

The nicest thing about this exercise is that, as a side benefit, you'll probably develop a deeper appreciation for the people you admire.

Activity: Phone a friend

Most of us value the opinions of our closest friends. This activity helps you to use your imagination to recruit them in your search for your values.

- Imagine I have the phone numbers of some of your closest friends. I phone them and ask them to describe what they like best about you.

- What would you like them to say?

- What would you hope they wouldn't say?

I love this one because I can imagine my friends responding to it. Some of them have a wicked sense of humour and they'd be likely to give some very funny answers. I also think the last question really helped me to clarify what matters to me.

The words I'd least like to hear used to describe me would include 'selfish' or 'mean'. This helped me to see that generosity and kindness are really important values for me.

I'd most like to be described with words like wise, giving, helping and creative.

Because our friends are people whose opinions are very important to us, this exercise can be a great way to home in on what really matters.

Activity: And the winner is…

Most of us enjoy events where we are acknowledged for our good works or achievements but if you don't like that kind of attention you may prefer to skip this one.

- You have won an award for something.

- What is the award for?

- What would you like to hear said about you when you are introduced at the presentation ceremony?

Some people love this one and others find it awkward. That's probably a reflection of different values around humility.

Of course my first thought is I would like to be handed an award for curing cancer, but I'm not a medical professional so this is a wish rather than a value.

An award for helping people recover from cancer is worth imagining, or perhaps an award for writing a really useful book!

I'd like to be described as 'generous' and 'dedicated to helping other people'.

Activity: Who you are not

This one reverses the previous strategies and gets you to think about the kind of behaviour you don't like.

- Think about the type of person you find annoying or frustrating.

- What is it about them that causes you to feel this way?

- What makes you angry about the behaviour of other people?

Thinking about what you don't value can help you to clarify what you do. This exercise can also give us some surprising insights into those aspects of our own behaviour that we'd like to work on.

I find people who monopolise a conversation annoying and yet I'm notorious for doing just that. It goes against my values regarding friendship and courtesy. My husband and I both hate it when someone talks over us, and we both do it all the time!

That's not to suggest that all the annoying behaviour I encounter is a reflection of my own. Sometimes it's a reflection of something that has happened in the past, or something I've observed in others that has had unhappy consequences.

For example, I also have strong values around people who falsely accuse others. I know this is connected to having been in the position of being falsely accused.

Taking some time to contemplate who you are not can yield some surprising insights into your values. If you loathe greed, dishonesty and cruelty it's reasonable to extrapolate generosity, honesty and kindness as important values. These are common values for most people and hardly a shock.

Realising that you feel angry when someone doesn't say thank you or that a failure to properly apologise for bad behaviour can leave you stewing for months is more interesting. Perhaps courtesy is a much more important value than you thought. Or perhaps you've uncovered some other important value.

Once again, be playful with this activity and don't get too caught up in past hurts or failures. It's a tool. Not a weapon.

Talking with friends and family

Discussions about values can be fun and very interesting.

I've had some great conversations with my husband, my daughter and my friends about which values we think are important.

Not surprisingly, the people close to me tend to have very similar values.

If you're struggling to do any of these activities on your own, consider discussing them with friends and family. You can use any of the activities as a starting point.

You might like to put the questions from these activities onto cards and take turns answering them. My husband and I have used this technique to strengthen our emotional intimacy and improve the quality of our communication. A question on a card doesn't come with the same trepidation that a direct question sometimes carries. The card has no subtext or hidden agenda. We can answer the question, or not.

Certainly spending time talking with anyone about what matters most can be a richly rewarding activity. It can also be a great way to help you clarify your own values.

A list of values

Still struggling? Here's a list of words commonly used to describe values. It's not the only list and you can find plenty of places online that offer you alternatives. There are even places where you can fill in a quiz to help you identify your values.

Or just work through this list and rate these words in importance from one to five, with one being 'not at all important' and five being 'really important'.

Acceptance
Adventure
Health
Helpfulness
Relationships
Mindfulness
Creativity
Intelligence
Passion
Personal growth
Professional achievement
Recognition
Authenticity
Caring for others
Family
Generosity and charity
Connection to other people, to nature or to animals
Gratitude
Love
Caring for the environment
Learning
Wealth
Kindness

Diligence
Sensuality
Animal welfare
Honesty
Balance
Bravery
Humour
Fun
Play
Leadership
Spirituality
Intimacy
Encouragement
Excitement
Fairness
Growth
Forgiveness
Tidiness
Cleanliness
Financial security
Safety
Making a difference.

Please feel free to add your own values if there's something missing for you. Then just score everything from one to five (with five being the most important to you)

Try not to get too bogged down with this. You're not setting anything in concrete. Some of the things on this list are very alike. This process works best if you do it quickly without agonising over it

Now take everything that scored a five (or everything that scored a four if you're one of those people who never scores a five) and write them on another piece of paper.

Now choose just five of those words. You're not excluding anything on the sheet of paper. You're just choosing which of your values are your top priorities right now. Don't overthink it. Nobody is going to judge you based on your answers and there's no one correct list.

Putting together your final list

How did you go? Did you find any of the activities particularly useful or was it simpler for you to work through the list? I've tried to give you a few different options because I know we all have variations in the way we figure out this sort of thing. Regardless of which method you used, it's time to see if you can narrow down your list to your five top values. Just like the last exercise, remember you're not leaving anything out. Most of us could create a list of 20 or more values.

Picking a top five is really about giving yourself a starting point for learning how to apply values-based living into your life. In the next section of the book I'll introduce you to some methods for doing this. Keeping the list to five will help. Having a list with too many values on it can leave you feeling swamped. This process should feel reassuring, not overwhelming.

Getting in touch with my values and learning how to apply them on a daily basis has given me a deep sense of satisfaction and contentment.

The last time I did this activity my list looked like this:

1. Health
2. Helpfulness
3. Mindfulness
4. Relationships
5. Creativity

Most cancer survivors have health as a very high value even if it wasn't when they were diagnosed so this was not at all surprising. It was interesting for me to see how high up the list 'helpfulness' came.

When I left the police force over a decade ago I was exhausted by helping others and I had avoided it. This exercise helped me to reconnect with this very important personal value.

It's not that I ever stopped helping people but I had become concerned about overdoing it. It's given me great joy and a sense of real purpose to return to helping other people while connecting it to one of my most important values.

Have a look back through your list of five. Is anything more important to you than you thought it would be? Are there any surprises on the list or is it pretty much what you expected.

My only caution with your top five is to make sure you've chosen things based on what you honestly value, and not on what you think might impress other people.

Remember, these are your personal values for where you are in your life right now. It could be you've spent a big part of your life helping others and now you've survived cancer you want to focus on adventure.

It could be that cancer made you realise you had spent far too much time pursuing wealth and status and what you really want to focus on now is helping other people. It might also be the case that your financial situation following treatment means that rebuilding wealth is a necessary priority.

You can see what I mean about values being very personal. Think of it as being a bit like choosing what you want in a restaurant. Everyone is there to eat but not everyone will order the same meal. The chicken isn't better than the fish. It's just a better choice for you.

What really matters is that your list is a good representation of your personal values.

If it helps you to clarify your values into sentences and you haven't already done that then you might like to take some time to rework them before moving on to the next section.

You're welcome to come back any time you like and reassess your values but try to focus on just five for at least a few months so you understand how to use them.

Think of your top five values as giving you a focus. Everything else is still there, in your peripheral vision, but these five are what you're going to give the most attention to over the next few months. All of your values represent what you want to stand for and these five are your most important right now.

Twisted values

Finally, here's quick word of warning about values. They are words that gently inspire you, not ropes that bind you. Here are some examples of the most common ways that people use their values to tie themselves up in knots:

If I don't do this I'm a bad person

I have to do this whether I like it or not

I should/must do that

This is the right thing to do

When I do this I'll impress people with how good I am

I don't think I can do this but I'm going to try.

Values are guidelines. There will always be times when, in spite of your best intentions, you act in ways that are inconsistent with them. Most of us have strong values around relationships with the people closest to us and all of us will, from time to time, act in ways that are not very kind or supportive. We are human. This is what we do.

Use your values to guide yourself back to the type of behavior you want to stand for.

Living a life consistent with your values doesn't make you better or more worthy than other people but it definitely makes you more comfortable with who you are. It also makes life consistently more enjoyable, even when awful things are happening to you or around you.

Living your best life

Welcome to the final step in overcoming your fear of recurrence.

By now you've hopefully had plenty of practice with taking a moment and noticing the difference between you and your thoughts. You've found some techniques for facing your fear and you've become proficient at using them when you need them.

You have figured out that your fear is not your enemy but a really useful emotion, just like all your other emotions. You now recognise there is no such thing as a negative emotion, just an uncomfortable one.

You've practiced acceptance, and being mindful and present in your everyday life, and you should have experienced a shift from your imagination pulling you in every direction, to an improved ability to be in the real world doing real things.

You have been introduced to the idea of values and you've spent some time identifying your top five. You know these are an expression of what really matters to you right now and what you want to stand for.

This section is about integrating your values into your life. I'm going to start with a simple technique to weave your values into how you deal with your fears around cancer. Then I'll move on to the big picture stuff.

Asking two questions about values

There are two simple questions that can help you to transform your fearful thoughts from something that is well managed to something that is beneficial

Is this thought useful?

Does this thought help me to live a life that is aligned with my values?

This is really the same question asked in two different ways. For our purposes, the definition of a 'useful' thought is one that helps you live a life aligned with your values. In time you will probably find you can drop the second question but I recommend leaving it in while you learn this technique. It reminds you that 'useful' has a very specific meaning.

You'll notice there's nothing here about whether or not a thought is true. There's no judging the evidence to support the thought and no attempt to rescript it in more appropriate language.

There's no classification of some thoughts as functional and others as dysfunctional and no arguing with yourself (as is required in some other methods of therapy).

You simply accept the thought in its original form, exactly as your mind presented it to you. It may well be an example of running a worst-case scenario, of black and white thinking or of attempting to predict the future. That's not what matters. Don't try to judge your thought. Just notice it and ask these questions.

What really matters is whether or not the thought is **useful**. I'll give you an example of how this works:

I get a text message reminding me I have a follow-up appointment with my oncologist. I feel frightened. My mind starts generating questions and statements about cancer.

I take a moment to do a quick reality check. I close my eyes, hold myself gently and take some calming breaths. I reconnect with my body and the world around me.

I face my fears by noticing my thoughts, and noticing myself noticing my thoughts. I might sing my fear to the tune of 'happy birthday'.

All of this helps me to separate out the emotion I am feeling from the person I am. I accept my fear is what it is, an emotion I am experiencing right now. I connect to the present.

Now I ask 'is this thought useful? Does it help me to live a life aligned with my values?'

Sometimes the thought isn't useful at all. When it isn't, I simply thank my mind.

'Thank you mind, for trying to keep me safe. I really appreciate it. But this thought isn't useful right now.'

Notice my tone. I'm not bullying myself or criticising my mind in any way. I just accept the thought and recognise it isn't useful to me right now.

Sometimes this is enough and the fear floats away, and sometimes my mind keeps on trying to scare me. If it does, I can use some of my other fear-facing strategies until I feel calmer.

Some frightening thoughts are very useful

Sometimes the thought is actually very useful. I'm going to show you what I mean by using that absolute champion of scary thoughts, one I think all of us have been terrified by at some point in time.

I am going to die!

I suspect it is impossible to get a cancer diagnosis without having this thought. It doesn't help to know that more people now survive cancer than die from it and, depending upon your diagnosis, you probably have a 50-80 per cent survival chance or better. We now understand why rationalising with our emotions and trying to rescript them doesn't help.

It's a thought we often keep to ourselves because we don't want to scare our loved ones.

It's a thought that can compound because once we start worrying about dying it's not uncommon to then worry about the impact the worry is having on our health. It doesn't help to dwell on whether or not this thought is true because, let's face it, sooner or later it will be. We really are going to die one day (but not today). Practicing acceptance helps us understand this.

So let's ask the question, **is this thought useful?**

I think it's a very useful thought. It reminds me to focus on what really matters. It helps me to let go of possessions, ideas, habits and even people that don't contribute to a fulfilling life.

Thinking about the possibility of my own death, when I turn and face it rather than running away from it, actually becomes one of the most useful things I've ever done.

I used to get ambushed by this thought. It would creep into bed with me at three in the morning and poke me with icy fingers. It would sneak up behind me and throw a bag over my head. Now we hold hands and play nicely together.

If you prefer, you can substitute the word **helpful**, but avoid worrying about whether any thought is reasonable, justifiable or even true. That's not what matters. A thought can be all of these things and still not be at all useful.

.

Activity: Is this useful?

Now here's an activity for you to try. Read all the way through it first and then come back and try it:

- Find somewhere to sit quietly and take a few deep, calming breaths.

- Remember the last time you were frightened of cancer returning. If you prefer, you can just start thinking about cancer and see what thoughts turn up.

- Breathe and make room for the thought to form into a clear sentence. So, if what comes up is fear, ask yourself what you are afraid of. If what comes up is anger, ask yourself what you are angry about.

- Now ask yourself if the thought is **useful**. Don't worry about whether it's true. That doesn't matter.

- If the answer is the thought is **not** useful, thank your mind for trying to keep you safe. You don't need to grab onto that thought. It's not useful.

- If the answer is that the thought **is** useful then ask yourself 'How is this thought useful?'

- You may want to write down a few notes about your useful thought or it may be enough to just think about it.

I think of this activity as finding treasure because it's been a rich source of great insights and the motivation that keeps me working towards being healthier. Here's another example:

I am in bed and about to drop off to sleep when I feel some nerve pain in my chest (this is very common for people who have had a mastectomy and feels a bit like broken glass or electricity). My mind has the thought 'the cancer is back'. It sounds like this:

THE CANCER IS BACK!

I breathe into the thought, make room for it and practice one of my activities for facing my fear. Then I ask myself if the thought is useful. I decide it's a very useful thought because it reminds me to do all the things I have promised myself I would do to stay healthy.

I use this thought as the motivation to regularly examine myself for any signs of recurrence, to keep my medical appointments and to avoid excessive alcohol consumption (because alcohol is a carcinogen).

I thank my mind for reminding me I once had cancer and for trying to help me to avoid getting cancer again. I use this process, and my other activities, to loosen the grip this thought has on me.

Sometimes the fear vanishes in a puff of insight and sometimes it looms like a rain cloud. It's all good. I know it will pass in its own time. I will not spend every remaining second of my life being frightened. It is what it is.

Of course, just because I find a thought useful doesn't mean you will. This particular thought, the fear of dying, cripples some people so badly that it sucks the joy from their lives. The thought is not at all useful.

It's still worth asking the question. Is this thought useful? If you don't find it useful just thank your mind for trying to keep you safe.

Please add this simple activity of asking if a thought is useful into your process for dealing with fear of recurrence and see what happens.

Remember, you can't learn to swim without getting in the water and you won't get any benefit from this activity without actually practicing it. The most common reason for not finding these methods helpful is not actually doing them. I'm yet to find anyone who has practiced them regularly without experiencing great results.

Practicing these techniques doesn't have to take up very much of your time. Five deep breaths and a bit of visualisation will usually take you less than five minutes. Most people can incorporate some thinking about usefulness into that five minutes and some enjoy taking a bit longer but, generally speaking, you're not going to need more than 10 minutes a day to regularly practice these techniques.

When something truly frightening happens, you will need to spend more time putting what you've learned into practice. That's okay because prior to learning all of this you probably would have spent the same amount of time, or longer, bound up in your own panic (I know I did).

I think of these questions as a kind of amplifier. Learning to take a moment and to face your fears are powerful techniques. They will work all on their own to help you deal with your fear of cancer returning. Practicing acceptance, and being mindful and present will help you to reduce both the frequency and intensity of your fears.

But adding in this last little bit is what flips everything from being a coping strategy to one that can greatly improve the quality of your life.

Activity: Values v fears

Here's an easy activity involving values that helps you to create a useful reminder of everything this book has taught you so far:

- Take a sheet of paper and on one side, write down all the scary thoughts you have about cancer. You might like to include the title you came up with earlier in this book. You can write a list or create a word map. It really doesn't matter what form the words take. You're just trying to create a visual representation of the stories your mind uses to scare you. (You might already have something like this in your back pocket.)

- Now turn the paper over and write down your top five values from the values activity. There's no magic about the number five. You can have more or less if you like.

- Sit comfortably. Turn the paper back over and hold it with both hands so close to your face that all you can see is the scary thoughts. Notice how when you do this you can't see anything else. You can't move from where you are. You can't kiss the people you love. In fact, you can't do anything at all.

- This is what it's like when your fear of recurrence grabs you and when you grab back. Take five deep, calming breaths.

- Now move the paper away from you. Lower it into your lap. Notice you can still see all of your scary thoughts but you can also see the world around you. Notice the room you are sitting in. Pay attention to the sights and sounds around you. Come back into your body and back into the present.

- Turn the paper over and look at your values. Think about what you can do today that will help you live a fulfilling life, consistent with those values.

- Notice all your scary thoughts are still on the piece of paper. You haven't thrown them away. Remember these thoughts are really your mind's way of trying to keep you safe. They can actually help you to remember to live a life according to what really matters to you.

- Fold up the piece of paper and put it in your pocket, or your wallet. The next time you find yourself feeling anxious about cancer returning, take out the piece of paper. Notice you've already made a really good record of the story your mind is trying to tell you (and you can add anything new that occurs to you). Reassure your mind that you get it; you understand the message. Thank your mind for trying to keep you safe.

- Turn the paper over again and look at your values. Think about what you can do today that will help you live a fulfilling life, consistent with those values.

At this point you might be happy to get rid of the piece of paper or you might like to carry it around indefinitely. Some people find this activity is a very useful and practical way of dealing with fear of recurrence. The paper is evidence you've paid attention. By taking it out and reading it, you are reassuring your mind the message has been received.

You don't need to hold the paper up to your face each time, but you can if this helps you to remember that grabbing onto your fear prevents you from living a fulfilling life.

Like all the activities in this book, you can play with this concept so it works best for you.

Most people find this activity really effective. It's as if you've said to your mind, "I hear you, and I thank you for the warnings, but I'm busy being connected to what really matters to me right now."

Unhelpful friends and healthy avoidance

Being clear about our values can be beneficial when we need to respond to unhelpful friends. This is another good skill to have in your toolkit. You're learning all these great new activities for dealing with your fear but your partner, children, parents and friends don't necessarily know much about them.

It might seem odd to them when you leave the room to sit quietly for a minute (but please do it anyway) and they may repeat things they've read or heard in an effort to be useful.

Remember, most people are genuinely trying to help you. Even the people who say really unhelpful things are not usually being mean or stupid on purpose.

My pet hate is the medical horror stories. I don't know why people think I would want to hear about someone else's cancer, or why these stories are so often about something going horribly wrong! I have become better at stopping these in their tracks, even though I have possibly caused some people discomfort when I do. Here's what I say as soon as I get an indication that a story is on the way:

It seems you're about to tell me a story about someone else's illness. I'm going to stop you there. I know you're trying to help but those stories really upset me.'

I would like to recommend you come up with your own version of this, using your own words. It's best to follow it up with some other suggested topic and the easiest thing is to get people to talk about themselves or someone close to them:

How about you tell me what your son has been up to lately?

I appreciate that, in many ways, this is a kind of avoidance but I think this is the healthy kind. We have enough real fears of our own without adding someone else's. It might be you're perfectly fine with these stories in which case feel free to discuss them.

It could be that what really annoys you is the unsolicited medical advice. This is often from the realm of alternative medicine or based on something people read on the internet. It's rarely a result of studying the research literature.

I find the easiest way to respond to this one is just to say this;

Thanks for that. I'll look into it.

On the rare occasion they follow up I usually say:

I really appreciate your concern but I don't think it's for me.

It's usually not worth getting into a discussion about the relative merits of any particular treatment, although I must admit I have done so when something particularly ridiculous is recommended. Just keep in mind that most people's intentions are good. They are genuinely trying to help and often struggling to know what to say. We can be grateful for that intention even if what they say is unhelpful.

I've seen lots of popular articles about what to say or not to say to people with cancer. I prefer to just be grateful that they are still in my life and appreciate that even what seems like the most obtuse comment can come from a good place.

Understanding values helps a lot with this. Different people have different values and their questions sometimes reflect this.

I still regularly get asked when I'm having breast reconstruction surgery. I'm not. I recognise the people asking the question have different values around breasts and reconstruction to me.

When friends behave in ways you find unhelpful it can be useful to recognise you may have identified a conflict in values. What motivates them is different to what motivates you. That doesn't make either of you wrong or right, just different. If you have a strong emotional reaction to that conflict you can make room for that emotion, name it and experience it, and then decide if you need to say anything.

But what if the cancer really IS back?

The techniques in this book are relatively easy to practice when all you're dealing with is a fearful mind, but what about those times when your body is the source of your fear?

For me this is twofold. On the one hand, I've had all kinds of weird pains and symptoms over the last few years. In addition to cancer, I have some arthritis and some aches and pains that come with age. Like most people, I sometimes get headaches or my body gets sore from extreme gardening. I still have nerve damage caused by treatment and nobody warned me that in a significant number of mastectomy patients there's continuing pain.

Once you've had cancer it is very common to fall into a habit of every single pain setting off alarm bells. Could it be cancer? Is it back? Worse still if you actually experience a cancer-related symptom like finding a lump. So what does it look like if you use these methods when you are dealing with physical symptoms?

First of all, take a moment. Breathe. Hold yourself gently and recognise the difference between you and the stories your mind is telling you. Use one of your favourite fear facing activities to give yourself room to experience your emotions without them overwhelming you. Use mindfulness to connect to the present.

Practice acceptance. It is what it is. If the cancer is back, then it's back. You won't know anything for certain until you have further tests. Pay attention to the way your fear feels and try an activity like clenching or unclenching.

Ask yourself if your fears are useful? Thank your mind for trying to keep you safe and recall your values. What do you want to stand for in this life, and in this particular situation.

You might like to practice some more mindfulness or meditation exercises to help you reconnect to the present and what matters to you. You might like to just think about your values and what you can do today that would be an expression of them.

Some people like to seek immediate medical help and some prefer to wait and see what happens with their symptoms. It's important to remember that avoidance is not your friend in situations like these. Waiting because a symptom is vague and not serious is very different to ignoring a lump because you don't want bad news. Connecting to your values around looking after your health will be beneficial right now.

The pain or lump might be cancer and it might not be. It is what it is. Being overwhelmed by fear will not be useful. You will need to have tests to determine if you need treatment. In the meantime you can use the methods outlined in this book to manage your fear. You are still going to be frightened. It would be inhuman not to feel fear when you have any concerns about cancer returning. It's also reasonable to expect your fear will require more time and effort if you're going to manage it well, but it can be managed.

Of course you don't need to find a lump or experience pain to become intensely fearful. Many of us have lingering doubts about our ability to identify cancer if it returns.

I had four tumors in my left breast that were undetectable without expensive medical equipment. If I had leant forward and looked back I would have noticed my naturally larger breast was now much larger, but I didn't notice this until I saw my MRI result. My tumours could not be felt through my skin. At the time of my diagnosis I would have told you I was in good health. This is why, for some of us, even those times when we have no symptoms can be a source of anxiety. Cancer snuck up on us.

I describe this as being like falling down a pit. I was walking along one day, living my life, when suddenly the ground opened up under my feet and I fell into this huge hole. I spent the next couple of years climbing out and it was not easy. Now I have a reasonable fear of it happening again, without warning.

You'll manage this type of fear much more easily if you get accurate information from your doctor about what kind of symptoms are likely to be cancer-related. It's helpful for me to know that if I do get recurrence, it will probably feel like a pea and it will also feel stuck to my chest wall. This helps, and I also continue to sometimes have free-floating fear in spite of an absence of symptoms.

I recognise that having fallen into a huge metaphorical pit my clever mind is now trying to keep me safe and to prevent that from every happening again. Thank you mind. The trouble is that I can't have any kind of life if I creep about, waiting for the earth to open up again. I'm also not going to avoid falling into a pit no matter how carefully I creep.

Dealing with this type of fear has been a major challenge. Unlike actual symptoms I can't get the reassurance of a doctor. All tests have associated risks and asking for a bone scan every time I feel an ache would be both dangerous and expensive. That is why the techniques in this book have been so valuable to me.

If you're in this situation, where you have free-floating fear of recurrence without any symptoms the protocol is the same. Start with taking a moment, then face your fears and add in some mindfulness to anchor you in the present. Practice acceptance. It is what it is. Ask yourself if your fears are useful. Do they help you to live a life more aligned with your values? Now connect with your values and ask yourself what you want to stand for in this particular situation and how you can live a life more aligned with what matters to you.

Some people report that, in spite of not having symptoms, they still want the reassurance of a visit to the doctor – and there's nothing wrong with taking that option.

Unlike many other forms of therapy that involve trying to reason with your irrational fears, these methods also work when your fears are genuine and perfectly reasonable.

I don't think it's helpful to re-script my inner dialogue when fear of recurrence strikes. I mentioned this type of strategy earlier. It often includes a list of all the wrong ways to think about something, including always looking on the downside of a situation, exaggerating the risks or dividing everything into black and white when you should recognise shades of grey.

You're encouraged to write down your 'automatic negative thoughts' and to rewrite them in a different format. This type of therapy definitely has benefits for some people in some situations but I think it's particularly useless when you're dealing with something like a potentially life-ending illness.

I used to be a fan of this kind of method and I became very good at re-scripting my inner dialogue. I hit a wall when my fears were legitimate. I also found this constant judgment of thoughts as 'functional' or 'dysfunctional' left me feeling damaged, as if my mind was somehow not working properly and I needed to be propping it up with analysis and logic. It felt as if my mind was creating monsters under the bed and I just needed to teach it not to be so stupid.

I'm not denigrating these methods. I acknowledge that they have helped many people live better lives and for many years I found them useful. I also found them hard work. Discovering an alternative to them was like discovering that my hands and feet had been secretly chained and that I had been carrying around the key. Learning to name my emotions and just ask if they were useful (rather than negative) had been both easy and enjoyable.

Notice there's nothing in the methods I've taught you that categorises any thought as negative or dysfunctional. It doesn't even matter if the thought is true. You just need to pay attention to the fear, recognise it as a story your mind is telling you (with all the best intention in the world) and ask yourself if the thought is useful or helpful. You are not being stupid, overreacting or being negative.

You then connect to the present and to your values. You do this gently, with kindness towards yourself and your mind. I know I've made this point before but it's so important, it's worth restating.

Learning these methods was a huge relief to me. My mind is doing what it is supposed to be doing. It does not need to be spoken to like a child having nightmares, bullied into submission, or labeled as broken.

I found that practicing these techniques when I've received really awful news has made a big difference to my ability to cope. When I received the news my cancer had returned, that it was active and invasive and that my breasts needed to be removed it was, in many ways, more terrifying than my original diagnosis.

My imagination went into overdrive. I was so sure I'd done everything to beat cancer, and so sure I had beaten it, that my mind didn't want to do anything except generate horror stories. The more I read about recurrence of my form of breast cancer the more convinced I became that I had only months to live. I was very, very frightened.

Facing my fears during this part of my life did not get rid of them. I didn't stop being seriously frightened until the pathology came back after my mastectomy with clear margins and no evidence of lymph node intrusion. While this reduced my fear it did not remove it.

I continued to be periodically frightened on a regular basis right up until the third anniversary of my diagnosis, where my statistical survival odds improved. While the frequency and intensity of my fears diminished with this important milestone, I still sometimes feel very frightened.

When things are really bad, fear is to be expected. I didn't find that these techniques banished my fear. What I did find was that by facing my fear I was able to live well in spite of it. I still feel fear, but I am free from the crippling effects of it.

I think the strength of these methods lies in how simple they are to apply, and the fact they work regardless of whether or not our fears are well founded. There is no way any amount of distraction, avoidance or trying to reason with myself would have helped me through this difficult time.

I found acceptance was particularly useful. I did not want to lose my breasts. The two weeks between receiving the diagnosis and having the urgent surgery included plenty of tears and fears. I made room for my genuine shock and grief, without judging myself. I found the phrase, 'It is what it is' both anchoring and calming. It was also very useful to name the waterfall of emotions that flooded through me. Here was anger, and grief, and frustration, and fear, and anxiety, and sadness. Here was acceptance, compassion, love and hope.

I don't know if I'll ever stop being frightened of the cancer coming back. I know it now happens less often, and that when it does happen it's less intense. I think the strategies in this book have been really useful tools for helping my brain to recover from the shock and fear of cancer.

If you haven't already done so, now would be a good time to review what you've read so far and to decide how much time you want to commit to doing this each day. You're also more likely to make it a habit if you can link it to some other regular daily activity.

If all you've done so far is to read about these techniques without practicing them, then please know you haven't started dealing with your fear yet. It's as if you have bought yourself some seeds, soil and pots, but you haven't actually planted anything. Nothing will grow without your effort.

So how are you going? I promised you something surprisingly easy and effective and hopefully you're experiencing what I meant by that. This stuff changed my life.

You might feel like you've learnt enough and you would like to take a break now. Feel free to do that. The next section moves on to some of the bigger picture stuff and I think it works best if you've become proficient at facing your fear. It's also a section best explored when you're not in the midst of treatment or frequently overwhelmed by fear.

If you're currently dealing with an actual recurrence, some frightening news or some symptoms that need tests, or if you've got anything else happening that is really holding your attention then put this book aside for a while or just use the information you've read so far to help you get through this. You have enough on your plate.

If you're ready to transform everything you've now mastered into a much more fulfilling life then please, read on.

Living a values-based life

So, connecting with your values is a great way to improve on your ability to deal with fear and anxiety. But wait, there's more.

I could have finished the book here. I've done everything I set out to do. I've passed along some great skills for facing your fears and living mindfully and by adding in a values component, I hope I've shown you how you can use your fears to improve your life. But I've found so much benefit in living a values-based life, even when I'm not fearful, I wanted to add just a little bit more.

First, here's a summary of what we now know:

Fear is normal and human and to be expected when you have had cancer

You are not crazy, or broken

Nobody is positive all the time and all healthy humans experience a full range of emotions

Experiencing a full range of emotions is part of the richness of life

Fear is a story your mind tells you to keep you safe (what a good mind!)

You can find ways to experience your fear safely, without it terrifying you

Acceptance can help you to effectively manage your reasonable fear

Being mindful and present allows you to appreciate and be grateful for all the good things in your life and to rebuild your brain

By being clear about what you genuinely value you can connect to what really matters to and live a more fulfilling life.

Living a values-based life is not just about responding to your fears. It's something you can do every day for the rest of your life. Outwardly, things might not look all that different. Inwardly it's likely to be a whole different story. All those revelations you had after cancer, about knowing what was important and what wasn't, about valuing your time and your life, become a much bigger part of your day when you connect to your values.

In particular I have noticed living a values-based life makes me much more appreciative of the things that most people would consider mundane. Dinner with my family, my weekly exercise class, coffee with friends and time in the garden are very 'every day'. Connect them to values and they are suddenly deeply meaningful activities.

I am certain that a focus on values is the missing link in a lot of self-help techniques. Mindfulness is useful, but if I'm mindfully doing something that is not aligned with my values I won't be fulfilled by it. Being present helps me to heal my brain and reduce my fears but that still leaves me with a whole lot of life to live. Values are the 'why' of life. Certainly a life without them feels like 'why bother?' or 'why not?'

Once you are clear about your values you can use them like a sailor uses a rudder. They will help you to take control of your life and steer it towards those places that matter most to you, regardless of how bad the emotional weather might be.

Without a clear understanding of what matters to you, you're just drifting and letting other people determine the course of your life. Once you are clear about your values, you can keep coming back to them. You can check in and ask yourself if your life is an expression of those values.

You will notice when you've drifted. It will become much easier to dedicate your time to the things that really matter and to happily avoid those that don't.

This last part is no small thing. Many of us spend our lives trying to please other people. There are others who seem to crave drama and conflict for its own sake, perhaps to give them some excitement in their lives. Neither is a fulfilling way to live.

Using your values as a guide will free you of the guilt that sometimes comes with saying 'no'. It will release you from meaningless conflict, where you find yourself fighting with someone over something trivial and can't remember how you got there.

It will allow you to surrender those expectations you collected from parents, teachers, friends and children, unless they genuinely align with your values.

A values-based life is a life well lived.

It may be that you have already figured this out. The next section will help you to determine if that's the case. It will also help you make changes if there's a mismatch between your values and how you are spending your time.

Activity: Useful questions about your values

Now you have a short list of your most important values, here's a list of questions to help you put your values into action.

- What is it about the way I currently live my life that reflects these values?

- What is it about the way I currently live my life that is inconsistent with these values? Why am I doing it?

- If someone who shared my values was describing me as 'inspirational', what behaviour would they describe?

- Is the way I treat other people consistent with my values and, if not, what needs to change?

- Is the way I spend my time aligned with my values or am I spending too much time on things that are not as valued?

- Looking back at the way I've spent my time over the last week, month or year, did my behaviour reflect my values? What would I do differently?

- What strategies could I put into place to live a life more closely aligned with my values?

These questions should help you to discover the opportunities around you for living your values. Do you need to join a gym? Start a group? Volunteer? Look for a different job? What is it about the life you are currently living that matches your values and what needs to change?

Most people also find a great deal of reassurance. This activity helps them to appreciate that a lot of what other people would consider mundane is actually deeply meaningful. I value order and cleanliness in my home and when I recognised this my chores became more enjoyable.

It could be you discover a lot of activities in your life that don't seem to reflect your values.

Sometimes just recognising this makes it easy to let go of them. Sometimes the task needs a bit more thought to make sure it isn't values-based. Asking why you're doing what you're doing can help.

Remember, your top five values are not your only values. You're just starting with five to practice the ideas you're learning.

Our values are complex, and vary depending upon the situation. It's okay to recognise a lesser value in some routine activity. You don't need to abandon anything that doesn't align with your top five.

Sometimes this activity causes people to rewrite their top five. Actually applying their values to real life helps them to realise some of the things they thought were important, really aren't (or vice versa).

I have one friend who was certain his financial wealth was a top value and when he looked at how he spent his time, and his money, he realised he already had a great life and enough financial security to retire. He's now happily involved in local arts organisations and is learning to paint.

Playing with your values is meant to be enjoyable and not a reason to beat yourself up. You are not a 'bad person' because you enjoy relaxation more than exercise, or financial security more than philanthropy. You are just a person, capable of both good and bad actions.

A caution here about blaming other people for things you don't like about your own life. This is not a map for ending a relationship. 'I value time alone and creativity therefore I need a divorce' is definitely jumping the gun. Having a conversation with your partner about values is a better starting point.

You might be surprised to learn they've also been feeling trapped or inhibited. This might result in both of you having activities apart or in doing more together, but please try this before you abandon anyone that isn't violent or abusive (them you should leave!).

Most of us are naturally inclined to live a life that is fairly closely aligned to our values. The difference with clearly identifying the link between what you do and what you want your life to stand for might be a fairly subtle one. Mostly what I've noticed is deep contentment.

Doing this exercise might also bring you to a place where you want to make some significant changes to how you spend your remaining time on earth. Values are great for making sure you move towards something meaningful, and don't make bad choices about the kinds of changes you choose.

Values also strengthen your commitment and make it much more likely that you'll succeed in achieving the changes that you want in your life. They boost motivation and link what you are doing to something that is deeply meaningful to you.

Accentuate the positive

So far I've written about using these methods to deal with what are commonly thought of as negative emotions. By now I hope I've made the case these emotions are healthy and normal and potentially very useful.

But what about those emotions usually regarded as 'good'.

It recently occurred to me that I could flip these techniques to make the most of emotions like joy and love and awe. I could use them to connect to the things I value deeply and to live a more fulfilling life.

Here's what that looks like for me:

When I notice myself experiencing a **pleasant emotion** I take a few deep breaths and come back into my body. I notice how I'm feeling and where the emotion seems to be located within my body.

I imagine myself expanding to allow that emotion to move through every part of my body. Then I imagine it beaming out of me like sunshine into the world.

I ask myself 'how is this useful?', which might seem like an odd thing to do, but it's given me some surprising answers. Usually it's something to do with reminding me of the things that really matter to me. It's always a reminder to do more of whatever got me feeling this way.

I then think about which of my values the emotion links to, because it always does. I was recently standing with my husband looking out over the ocean and thinking about how easy it is to be happy in his company. It's the same when I'm at a yoga class or enjoying healthy food with friends.

I have always enjoyed these activities but reflecting on how they are connected to what really matters to me has made life much more fulfilling. It's interesting to me that these changes are just about how much attention I give something. Everything else is much the same as it always was.

Connecting what I'm doing to my values also helps me to be more present and mindful.

I call this process 'savouring'. It's a bit like that thing we do when we taste something really delicious and we take the time to focus on everything about the flavour and texture of it.

I've found taking time to savour the joyful aspects of my life has made me generally a more contented person. You might like to try it too. Savouring can be particularly powerful when we've identified those things that help us to achieve a state known as 'flow'.

Wonderful distraction and going with the flow

You probably recall earlier on in this book I took a big swing at strategies that rely on distraction to help us cope with fear of recurrence. I also mentioned at there were some notable exceptions.

All of us have something that puts us into a state known as **flow**. You know what these activities are because if you're not careful, time gets away from you. You find yourself so completely caught up in what you're doing that it's possible to skip a meal or forget and appointment.

Some of us are fortunate enough to have a few different flow activities. I find gardening and painting both do it for me. My mind is completely engaged in either activity. This is very different to trying to distract myself from fearful thoughts. In fact, I find it very difficult to start gardening or painting while I'm feeling frightened, so I'll usually take a moment to soothe myself.

Depending upon my fear level, I might also use some of my fear-facing techniques. Then I can head out into the garden or break out the watercolours and totally immerse myself in something I love.

There's a subtle but important difference here. I'm not gardening to take my mind off cancer. I'm gardening for its own sake, because I love it. I think using something you love to take your mind off cancer can backfire; you can end up associating something you used to love with cancer.

Research into flow activities has found they are invariably things we find challenging, but not too challenging. They play to our natural strengths and align with our values. There's no limit on the type of activity that puts you into flow. For some people it's a kind of sport. For others it's creating or repairing something.

I have a good friend who finds cleaning out her kitchen cupboards extremely satisfying and totally engaging (if only she felt that way about my kitchen cupboards!). My point is that it doesn't matter what puts you into flow. Just find something that does.

I would recommend that if you are feeling fearful, you still use taking a moment and facing your fear as your preparation. It's also good to get in touch with your values. Often the answer to 'is this thought useful?' turns out to be related in some way to doing things you really enjoy.

Knowing what your flow activities are is very beneficial when you need to fill a stretch of time, like the lead-up to surgery or the wait for test results. It helps time fly while giving you something to do that is genuinely rewarding. It's easy for me to go with the flow once my mind knows I'm paying attention to its very sensible warnings.

Being in flow has also been shown to be useful in dealing with chronic pain and depression, but these are side benefits. Always remember you should seek out flow activities for their own sake.

Flow is worthwhile at any time. It's a physical expression of what really matters to us. The more time we can find for the activities that put us into flow, the more closely we are connected to whatever it is that brings us deep satisfaction. The truly fortunate among us are those who have found a way to connect their flow activity to earning income. These people love what they do for a living.

Setting goals using your values

So now you have a short list of your top values and some ideas about how you might make a few changes. A lot of those might be fairly simple. You might decide to stop doing something that isn't aligned, or to spend a bit more time doing something that really matters. You probably won't need to do much more than simply make a decision and start living that change.

But there are other changes that benefit from a bit more structure. These tend to require more time and effort. If you're having difficulty shifting from where you are to where you want to be then here's a great technique for forming those ideas into achievable goals.

Activity: SMART goal setting

You might have previously seen something called SMART goals. (I don't usually like acronyms but this one is worth learning.) I've played with this model a little to align it to living a values-based life. I have also put it into an activity so you can get some real practice.

Pick one of your top five values. I'm going to use 'health' for this exercise because everyone I've met who has come out the other side of cancer has this as one of their top five. Now you're going to put together a clear statement about improving your health.

Goals like this are often overwhelming. Relax. You're not going to ask you to set a goal for everything to do with your health.. Just choose something you would like to change. It might be that you want to get more exercise, improve your diet or drink less alcohol. All of these are already goals but research into human behaviour suggests you'll be more likely to actually achieve them if you use something called the SMART model.

Choose a health related activity and see if you can write yourself a goal statement using this format:

- **Specific** – it's clear about what you are hoping to achieve rather than being vague.

- **Measurable** – there's a target you can actually measure to know you've achieved it.

- **Aligned with values** – (This one usually reads 'achievable' but I think 'realistic' has that covered so I've changed it.) A goal that's aligned to your values will contribute to a more fulfilling life. You will also be much more motivated to achieve it.

- **Realistic** – There should be a reasonable prospect of achieving the goal, given your current abilities and resources.

- **Time bound** – SMART goals have a finish date or a time schedule, so you commit to achieving something by a particular point in time or to doing something on a regular basis.

An example of a SMART goal would be something like this:

I will attend two yoga classes every week for the next six months in pursuit of better health. This is specific. I'm going to attend two more yoga classes every week. It's measurable because I can count those classes and record how often I attend. There is an obvious alignment with my values around being healthy and it is certainly realistic. Putting a six month limit on it makes it time bound and provides me with an opportunity to review my progress. At the end of six months I might want to add another class, or try something different.

Can you see the difference between a SMART goal and 'do more exercise'? One is a vague intention and the other is a clearly stated goal.

The next thing to do is to take action towards achieving your SMART goal. The sooner you do this, the more likely you are to stick with it. For my example, I joined a gym with a good yoga teacher, bought a mat and some yoga gear and put the two classes on my calendar for the next six months.

All these preliminary steps made it much more likely I would manage to attend two yoga classes a week for six months. In fact, seven years later I'm still going to class and I now practice yoga every day at home.

Not all goals are SMART

There are a few pitfalls with SMART goals. The main one is around what is actually realistic. As an example, it's realistic for me to set a goal to practice yoga for at least five minutes every day but it's not realistic for me to set a goal to teach yoga within six months, because teacher training takes longer than that and I'm not yet experienced enough to teach.

The trouble is some people sabotage themselves by being certain they can't do something before they even try. As an example, I read some work on rebuilding neural pathways in my forties and decided to learn a musical instrument. Because my husband, a musician, recommended I learn something I loved, I chose the cello.

I didn't know learning the cello was really difficult compared to something like the piano.

A cello is fretless, which means you need to learn to hear when a note is correct whereas you can just hit the right note on a piano. If I had known this I may never have pursued cello playing.

I also encountered people who wondered why someone my age would want to learn an instrument at all, or viewed it as somehow indulgent or mildly eccentric.

I am not a natural musician. Even so, I taught myself to read music and to play the cello well enough that the cats didn't run from the room!

My cello is a private pleasure and learning it is consistent with my values. It's helping me to rebuild my brain. It's also giving me a great deal of pleasure and a sense of achievement. Apart from my daughter's 18th birthday party I have never played to an audience. That was never my goal.

I'm often surprised by the lists people have of the things they can't do. 'I'm not good at organising things,' says one friend. 'I'll always be hopeless with numbers,' says another.

It's as if they are describing things they can't change, like their height. Why do we categorise ourselves like this? Who told these people they couldn't do these things? It's not as if simple organisational skills or basic maths are particularly hard to learn.

My view is that if another capable human being can do it, then anyone can learn to do it. We may not do it as well as someone else, but we can certainly achieve a reasonable level of competency if we're prepared to put in a bit of time and effort.

Other people with functioning brains and working hands play the cello. Therefore it's possible for me to play the cello. The variables, including my age, dexterity and musical ability, will influence how well I will be able to play but not whether I can learn.

Even some degree of mild disability is only a limiting factor, and not a reason to quit. Chemotherapy gave me peripheral neuropathy in my hands and my scar tissue means I had to learn to hold the cello differently.

This is just like everything else in my life. In everything I ever do there will be those who do it better and those who don't. The brilliance of Yo-Yo Ma is not a reason to never learn the cello. He's a reminder of the amazing things a dedicated human being can achieve when hard work and natural ability are combined.

Excellence in others should inspire us, not discourage us from even trying. What if instead of *I'm not good at...*we could only choose between *I'm not yet good at... 'or I choose not to be good at...?*

So when it comes to being realistic, what matters is doing something to the best of **your** ability. Be happy to head in the direction of your goal and just as happy to change course if things don't work out. You'll still be travelling and moving through your adventurous life. The other trap with SMART goals is assuming that because you can link it to a value it is necessarily a good idea.

For example, you might think deciding to have sex with your partner twice a week is a good way to pursue the value of 'connection' or 'increased intimacy', but if that goal leaves you feeling obligated and results in you feeling less like sex then it's not a worthwhile goal. Be prepared to abandon anything that isn't working.

My advice is to start with something that is closely aligned to one of your most important values, because this will ensure you are strongly motivated to achieve it, and to start small, because this will ensure you are more likely to succeed. If your value is helping the environment then you might want to start with reducing your own waste rather than taking down the coal companies.

Here's a popular example of starting small. Let's say you want to lose 16 kilos. Which of the following goals do you think will be more motivating:

I will lose sixteen kilos

In pursuit of better health I will lose two kilos in the next three weeks by following the 5:2 diet (you can insert your preferred diet plan here)

I will give up wheat, sugar and dairy.

What is your emotional response to each of these goals? What is your clever mind telling you about them? Most people find the second one feels reasonably achievable. They also find that in response to the other two, some part of their mind says something like this:

You know that's not happening!

Or this:

Oh here we go again with the whole dieting torture. As if that's ever worked!

Of course you now have the skills to respond to these thoughts. You can make room for them, ask yourself if they are useful and thank your mind for trying to help you to avoid disappointment, and this will help you realign with your goals in any similar situation, but how much easier to choose a goal where your mind responds like this:

Two kilos. I can do that.

SMART goals are great. They help you to turn something like 'I want to be healthier' into specific plans of action. But they are not the only kind of goal and not everyone enjoys using them. This is only a tool. In some cases, it is a tool that's far too big for the job. Some goals are simple to identify and easy to implement. For things that need a little bit more planning you might find SMART goals useful and it's also fine if you prefer to take a more organic approach.

Soft systems

SMART goals appeal to people who like to be clear and specific about where they are going. They have their rudder down and they know their desired destination. But a fulfilling life isn't always about getting somewhere. For some, it's more about enjoying where they are.

Soft systems are those that don't necessarily have a starting point and an end point. A really good example of a soft system is a garden. You pay attention to your environment, choose some plants, make some improvements and you have a garden, but you're never 'done'.

Over time, some things grow and create shade. Other things spread and thrive. Your expertise grows along with your plants. Some things die and you decide not to grow them again. You learn about plants with short life cycles and those that will live for many years after you've gone.

Your garden might be a source of food, medicinal plants, flowers or honey. It might be a habitat for wildlife or a private sanctuary. You might grow it to add value to your home, to provide a play area for your children or to give yourself a creative outlet.

Some people prefer to approach their lives in a similar way.

Being clear about your values will still be hugely beneficial if this is your approach to life. You will probably have things like creativity, flexibility, spontaneity and continuous learning on your list (which is not to say that lovers of structure and SMART goals will not). You would probably prefer to just put your goals on display somewhere and imagine different possibilities for a while.

You'll then start planting some of your ideas to see what grows. You'll be relaxed about abandoning something that doesn't seem to be working. You might have some activities you only do for a few months or a few years before moving on to something else.

If you're a soft systems kind of person, having clear values is like having really good soil in your garden. You're going to be able to grow a lot more of what really matters to you.

Here's one example of what this might look like:

Put your top five values on a large sheet of paper, somewhere towards the middle.

Start drawing lines out from each value and writing in ideas for things you could do that would turn that value into action.

Put your values poster on display somewhere.

Schedule time each week to do something from the poster.

You can be even looser than this if you like. Just put your top five values on display somewhere and check back daily, weekly or monthly. Think about what you've done recently in pursuit of them and what you're planning to do in the near, middle and distant future. Write in a journal or make art about your values.

Stay alert for opportunities to live your values. Use your values to make decisions about what you will do, and what you can comfortably decline. You're allowed to stay open and flexible to anything that comes up. They're your values and this is your life.

Sometimes a combination of SMART and soft approaches works best. Play with your own values and figure out what works for you.

The really, really big picture

I hope this last part of the book has given you some ideas for turning your values into action. Start doing this (if you haven't already) and you'll find life becoming increasingly fulfilling and meaningful. If you'd like to amplify this effect then you'll enjoy this section.

Not all goals are about achieving things in the short, medium or longer term. There's also the type of goals that are about each of us deciding what we want our life to stand for. These are the really, really big picture goals. This is the 'what I want my obituary to say' stuff. It's about your legacy, and how you want to be remembered.

You probably did some thinking around this while you were figuring out what your top values are. Here are a few different examples of other people's big picture goals:

I want to be remembered as someone who was a good and kind person, who made a difference in the world and left it a better place than I found it.

I am creative. I am drawn to all kinds of creativity and I love to make beautiful things. I also love to inspire, move and confront people with my art. I want my art to live on after I am gone and for it to continue to move people emotionally.

I am passionate about the environment and the protection of the natural world. I would like to be remembered for that, and for all of my environmental activism. I want to live my life in a way that has as little impact on the planet as possible.

I came from a background where we could never be sure of anything. My purpose has been to provide my family with emotional and financial security. I never want them to suffer the anxiety I experienced. I've also dedicated time and money to helping other people from disadvantaged backgrounds.

I'm an engineer. I turn ideas into real things. They are well built and safe. This gives me a lot of satisfaction. I'd like to be remembered for that, and for always being a good person.

I want to be famous and to have a huge funeral where all my fans are weeping. I want to be known as one of the finest bass guitarists on the planet!

You can see from these examples that the big picture stuff will always be connected to personal values. This is a virtuous circle. Being clear about your values helps you to connect to your life's purpose and being clear about your life's purpose helps you to connect to your values.

People who are feeling as if their life is pointless or meaningless can be rejuvenated by some time spent reflecting upon what really matters to them, and what they want their life to stand for.

Have a look back through your life so far. How would you describe it? What patterns and themes keep emerging? Has your life been a reflection of your values? It's never too late to connect to something fulfilling.

Some people will blame luck or poor circumstances on their apparent inability to live a fulfilling life, and yet we can see evidence all around us of people who have emerged from the most appalling circumstances to lead rich and rewarding lives.

I've met people who have survived war, disability, injury, chronic illness, domestic violence and child abuse. Some of these people believed they were permanently damaged and broken. Others did not. That single decision, to see themselves as either capable of living a fulfilling life or incapable of living a fulfilling life, had more to do with the quality of their life than anything else.

What I've noticed since learning these techniques is that the thriving survivors all had a strong connection to their personal values and the belief that it was possible to use them as a compass for their life. They also excelled at acceptance and being present and mindful. The past was gone. It only existed as imperfect memories in their heads. They could let it go.

I've been particularly inspired by some of the teenagers I met working in child protection. In spite of common expectations that they would be permanently damaged by what must be one of the most horrific experiences anyone can imagine, they overcame their trauma. I remember all of them. They are deeply inspirational to me.

I take nothing away from the fact that many of these teenagers were supported by committed professionals, including social workers, police, psychologists, doctors and therapists. My point is that however they managed to achieve a rich and fulfilling life, they proved that it was possible. Regardless of our personal circumstances, we always have the opportunity to rethink our values and change our direction. There's help available if we need it.

Please consider using what you've discovered about your values to improve your sense of fulfillment and contentment. It's not necessary to radically change every aspect of your life. Start small. Choose something challenging but achievable and pursue that. Build on your success to move onto something a bit more challenging. Keep going.

This approach mimics the formula used to design highly successful computer games. It's a proven way to harness your own powers of motivation. Remember, most of us really don't enjoy doing nothing. It's human nature to enjoy something that stretches us, challenges us and leaves us with a sense of accomplishment.

The key here is to divide things into levels that are challenging, but not so difficult that we doom ourselves to disappointment. The weight loss example I used earlier did this. By focusing on losing just a few kilos rather than a final goal weight you can break a task down into achievable chunks.

The other valuable lesson from game design is the safety to fail. Play any of these games and you soon realise the only way to develop expertise is to fail over and over and over again. The game restarts. You try again. Fear of failure cripples so many people. Those that see failure as a learning opportunity overcome this.

When you start heading off on your values-based adventures, please remember to be kind to yourself. Learning and changing usually involves mistakes. They're an opportunity to learn and improve. Aim for improvement rather than perfection.

This is the other advantage of breaking your big picture goals into smaller bits. If you fail at anything it's just a small part of the whole. You'll hopefully have already stored away some brownie points for yourself by the time this happens so reflect on your past successes, figure out what went wrong if you can, and have another go.

Remember that Einstein said stupidity is doing the same thing and expecting a different result (which at the very least should reassure us that even one of the greatest geniuses that ever lived was familiar with failure!) If something isn't working then don't just go back and try what you've already tried. Come at it from another angle.

Some people tell me they are much too busy to add anything new to their life. I ask them what they are busy doing and invite them to stack this activity up against their values.

If you've checked your life against your values and found things are nicely aligned, I'd recommend you just keep doing whatever you have been doing (and congratulations, you're among a very small group of people). If, however, your life is ruled by obligations and meeting other people's expectations then it's probably time to reassess what really matters to you.

If you're feeling really stuck then it can help to remember the great lessons cancer taught you. Life is finite. This is not a dress rehearsal. Time is precious. Do what really matters to you.

There's still a fair amount of stigma attached to getting help from a psychologist for most people. I don't know why. They are a great source of support and advice. If you're feeling stuck and you have the opportunity to see a professional then I highly recommend it. This entire book came about because I was introduced to Acceptance Commitment Therapy during my treatment. If you like the methods described in this book, then look for an ACT trained therapist.

Life without goals

Not everything in life needs to be done in pursuit of a goal. I don't think you'd have much of a life if you did this exclusively, but there are whole chunks of life that benefit from being uncertain, from being open to interesting possibilities and from letting circumstances take you to unexpected places.

Sometimes our goals can be self-limiting. Sometimes we can be so focused on achieving something we forget about all of those activities that aren't goal focused. It can be fun and interesting to let chance, circumstance or other people direct our lives from time to time.

I appreciate that 'letting go' or 'being creative' might actually be goals but there's also something to be said for just waiting to see where the day takes you. Good luck is often just the ability to recognise an opportunity. If all we can see are our goals we can sometimes miss the unexpected.

It's also essential to understand the importance of play. As children we all play naturally. As adults we tend to disregard most play as unimportant, unless we can link it to some kind of goal. But the point of play is to play! We should pursue play for the joy of it, for its own sake. If you've fallen out of the habit then try making a list of the things you used to love to do as a child, and as a teenager. (Perhaps limit this to the healthy things you did as a teenager!) This can reconnect you to things that bring you joy.

So I'd recommend you balance your goals-based activities with some that are not directly goal focused. Sit on the beach and watch the sun come up. Talk for hours with a good friend. Curl up with a book by the fire in winter. Entertain your dog or cat for an hour with whatever game they want to play. Let a child host a tea party with bears and you as the guests.

When your mind tells you that activites like this are pointless, or a waste of time, thank your mind and do them anyway, for the sheer joy of it.

Play and being open to whatever the day offers you can both be good for your mental health, great opportunities for connection with others and perhaps linked to your values in other ways, but I'd suggest some aspects of our lives are better lived more lightheartedly than that. Just have fun.

Whatever kind of goal setting you choose to do, it should be a source of inspiration rather than a rod for your own back. These models are meant to help us live better lives, not to punish us with unreasonable deadlines and harsh expectations. We should set our goals gently.

It's also good to remember that we've been through a period of time when it was enough to just get through the day. And the world did not fall apart without us. Somehow, everything that needed to get done still got done. Or it didn't, and that was fine too.

Perhaps one of the risks of recovery is that we'll try to play catch up, or we will be so mindful of the limited nature of life that we'll try to cram in as much as possible. Getting the balance right can be a challenge. I think that's why taking the occasional day to just see where life takes you can be so beneficial.

I am deeply grateful I'm able to finally make plans for the future again. I've set some big goals and some SMART steps to achieve them. I'm also remembering to stop and smell the roses.

And finally

Well that's about it for now. Thanks for staying until the end. I hope this book has given you some really simple and easy strategies for improving your life.

If you've done the activities as you went along you're probably only spending about five to 10 minutes each day practicing them but you're seeing great big improvements in return.

You should now have practical skills for each of these categories:

Take a moment

Face your fear

Acceptance (hold hands with the monster)

Be present and mindful

Find your focus

Living your best life

You might just use the activities from one section on their own, or in a different combination. Feel free to play with what works for you. The most important thing is you find yourself increasingly relieved of that crippling and distressing fear that is part and parcel of recovering from cancer.

You might also have added in another five minutes or so once a week to record the things you're grateful for. If so, you're probably noticing this is transforming your state of mind to a consistently more optimistic one.

Bonus points if you've also set aside a bit of time to practice meditation. You might have incorporated this into your daily activity for getting back into your body. I do. It's fine to do both together. Or perhaps you've found ways to be more mindful and present without meditation. That will benefit you too.

Please know these techniques work. They have worked for me and for thousands of other people. All I've done is to put them into a format that I hope makes them relevant to cancer survivors.

These techniques always remind me of the shift I experienced towards dandelions when I discovered they were a potentially cancer-thwarting food. Up until then I had always considered them weeds. In the same way, I used to regard my fear as weakness, failure and some kind of dysfunction of my mind. Now I know my fear is evidence of my mental health and a source of opportunity to connect to what really matters to me.

I hope you've also had the opportunity to use your work with values to move towards living a more fulfilling life.

If you've enjoyed this book and found it helpful then please spread the word. My main motivation for writing it was to help other people who have been through cancer treatment and struggled, as I did, with recurring fear. Feel free to leave a review, post a link somewhere or just pass it on to someone else.

Finally, my very best wishes for your continued recovery. Never doubt that life can be rich and fulfilling and wonderful after cancer.

Mine is. Yours can be too.

Gratitude

I know it's traditional to put acknowledgements at the beginning of a book but, honestly, who reads them?

If you've come this far then **thank you**. I am grateful that you enjoyed the book enough to see it through to the end. I'm a self published author, which is code for not having any money to do any sort of advertising, so I'd be even more grateful if you could pass this book on to someone else.

To finish things in a way that's consistent with my own values, here is a small example of my deep gratitude to all those that helped bring this book to life.

Thank you to Liz Swanton, a dear friend and professional writer who helped me to believe I was capable of writing a book and who spent many hours giving me the benefit of her considerable wisdom.

Thank you to Kerry Wagland, the psychologist that introduced me to ACT. Who knew that just two sessions with you could have such a profound impact. I am deeply grateful to you.

Thank you to Russ Harris for his wonderful books 'The Happiness Trap' and 'The Reality Gap'. I highly recommend both. Thanks also to the entire ACT community for your generous open source approach to this knowledge. There is no upper limit to how useful it can be.

Thank you to all of the amazing medical professionals that have cared for me over the last four years. The Gosford BreastScreen team, My GP, Dr. Hiew, Dr Kylie Snook and her patient advocate, Louise Cutts, Dr Rachel Dear, Dr Andrew Fong and their respective teams, and to the wonderful staff at the Mater Hospital, North Sydney and the Mater Imaging centre. I am alive to write because of all of you.

Special mention to the Breast Care Nurses and a heart felt wish that our health system finally comes to appreciate the enormous support you give patients and the extent to which you free up doctors from endless patient inquiries. You deserve to be paid accordingly and patients deserve to have access to you, no matter where they are in the country. You should be fully government funded and not dependent upon charity donations. Rant over.

Thank you to Emma Spivey, my gifted and generous yoga teacher, for creating a space of safety and healing, even when I was bald or burnt or lacking decent immunity or was recovering from surgery. Your gentle wisdom is woven throughout this book in the same way it is now a part of every healthy cell in my body. You were correct. Just five minutes of yoga every day did change my life. I am grateful beyond words. Namaste.

Thank you to everyone in the Thursday yoga class that made me feel so welcome with special mention to Trish, Gayl, Sharon, Jaki, Nicksta, Helen, Jan and Mike and to friends near and far for all your love and support.

Thank you to Maryanne Losurdo for all the oncology massage and the genuine healing that comes with it. You are a key factor in my survival and my wellness. I am grateful for you wisdom and your friendship.

Thank you to all the people that supported my blog and sent me their encouraging comments. Special mention to those who loved my writing and told me, many times, not to give up, particularly David, Ricki and Michelle. This book was inspired by all of you.

Thank you to Mum for fiercely refusing to accept the possibility of my early demise and for all your support. I love you.

Thank you to my other parents, Bill and Thelma, for their generous love and advice. I love you both.

Thank you to my wonderful husband, Graham, who continues to exceed all reasonable expectations. I really don't think I'm a genius, but it's a huge advantage to share my life with someone that believes I am. You are my best friend. I love you.

Thank you to Zoe, my inspirational daughter. I'm so sorry for everything you had to endure because I had cancer and so grateful that it didn't stop you from achieving your own goals. You are braver and stronger than most people I know. Thank you for encouraging me to share the good that came out of this whole, awful experience with others. I love you to the moon and back.

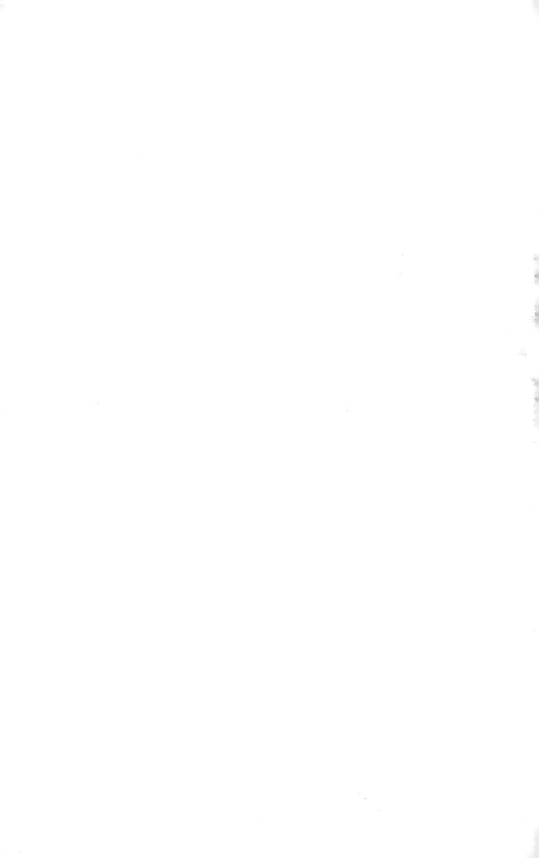